Caring for Dying Children and Their Families

Edited by

Lenore Hill

Head Nurse
Martin House,
Clifford,
Wetherby,
UK

Illustrations by
Helen Scouller

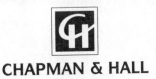

CHAPMAN & HALL

London · Glasgow · Weinheim · New York · Tokyo · Melbourne · Madras

Published by Chapman & Hall, 2–6 Boundary Row, London SE1 8HN

Chapman & Hall, 2–6 Boundary Row, London SE1 8HN, UK

Blackie Academic & Professional, Wester Cleddens Road, Bishopbriggs, Glasgow G64 2NZ, UK

Chapman & Hall GmbH, Pappelallee 3, 69469 Weinheim, Germany

Chapman & Hall Inc., One Penn Plaza, 41st Floor, New York NY 10119, USA

Chapman & Hall Japan, Thomson Publishing Japan, Hirakawacho Nemoto Building, 6F, 1-7-11 Hirakawa-cho, Chiyoda-ku, Tokyo 102, Japan

Chapman & Hall Australia, Thomas Nelson Australia, 102 Dodds Street, South Melbourne, Victoria 3205, Australia

Chapman & Hall India, R. Seshadri, 32 Second Main Road, CIT East, Madras 600 035, India

Distributed in the USA and Canada by Singular Publishing Group Inc., 4284 41st Street, San Diego, California 92105

First edition 1994

© 1994 Chapman & Hall

Typeset in 10/12 Palatino by Mews Photosetting, Beckenham, Kent
Printed in Great Britain by Clays PLC, Bungay, Suffolk

ISBN 0 412 47720 3   1 56593 135 1 (USA)

A catalogue record for this book is available from the British Library

Library of Congress Catalog Card Number: 93-74210

Contents

iv   *Contents*

Contributors

Sue Alder RGN RSCN Symptom Control Team, The Hospital for Sick Children, Great Ormond Street, London, UK

Sharon Beardsmore RGN RSCN Symptom Control Team, The Hospital for Sick Children, Great Ormond Street, London, UK

Michael Brady MRCGP Martin House Children's Hospice, Clifford, Wetherby, UK

Elizabeth Bryan Paediatrician, The Multiple Births Foundation, Queen Charlotte's and Chelsea Hospital, London, UK

Jack Cadranell Clinical Psychologist, St James' Hospital, Leeds, UK

Angus Clarke Senior Lecturer in Medical Genetics, Institute of Medical Genetics, University of Wales, Heath Park, Cardiff, UK

Janet Goodall Retired Paediatrician, Stoke on Trent, UK

Mark Hayter Nurse Tutor, School of Advanced Nursing Studies, Lodge Moor Hospital, Sheffield, UK

Hugh J. Heggarty Paediatrician, York District Hospital, York, UK

Lenore Hill Head Nurse, Martin House Children's Hospice, Wetherby, UK

Celia Hindmarch Freelance Counsellor, Former Manager of The Alder Centre, Royal Liverpool Children Hospital, Alder Hey, Liverpool, UK

Elizabeth Hopper Counselling Sister/Midwife, St George's Hospital, London, UK

Michael Kavanagh St Nicholas Vicarage, Beverley, E. Yorks, UK

Jean Lavelle Retired Special Needs Liaison Teacher, Leeds, UK

Jane Thomas Bereaved parent, Worcester, UK

Contributors

Tessa Wilkinson Former Bereavement Visitor and Member of Care Team at Helen House Hospice, Oxford, UK

Linda Zirinsky Lecturer in Child Psychiatry, The Royal Free Hospital, Hampstead, London, UK

Preface

The contributors to this book have been privileged to share, to some extent, in the lives of families where a child, or children, have died. Each chapter deals with a particular aspect of care, but because it is very difficult to look at any aspect in isolation some topics are covered in more than one chapter. As readers may wish to use only chapters relevant to a particular situation, it seemed right to allow these areas of overlap.

For ease of reading 'he' has been used throughout the book, but all the points made are just as applicable to either sex.

Those of us involved with the families of dying children must respect the wishes of the children and the families we seek to serve. Their fears, anxieties and needs must be listened to, and they must be allowed to stay in control of decisions. They will want, as far as is possible, to maintain some normal family life. If we are sensitive to these things then it may be that we will help to ease the burden a little. If not, our involvement may add to their burden. Families may be left with regrets and bitterness that were avoidable.

To lose a child suddenly or as the result of a long and debilitating illness is an overwhelming experience for families. From the time of first hearing the bad news, lives are irrevocably changed. After the death, parents, brothers and sisters, and others who have loved the child, slowly come to the realization that their child has gone forever. They will never again hold their child, feel his hair in their fingers, or hear his giggle.

Those of us involved with families during these traumatic years must never forget that this is **their** experience which we cannot live for them. We must be sensitive to differences in family ethos and culture and not impose upon them ours and society's feelings of right and wrong in the choices they may be compelled to make.

There is a cost to being alongside these children and their families, and we will need to find support for our grief too. There is also a lot to be gained if we are brave enough to be truly open and vulnerable in our relationships with them. These children never leave unchanged the lives they have touched.

Acknowledgements

I would like to thank all the contributors for sharing their experience. Special thanks to Jane Thomas for being willing to share her own and her family's experiences with Archie.

Thank you to Robin Wood for his help and advice and to Sue Wigley for deciphering and typing the manuscript. Thanks also to all the staff of Martin House for their patience during the production of this book.

The biggest thank you of all goes to the children and families who have enriched our lives by sharing theirs with us.

And can it be that in a world so full and busy the loss of one weak creature makes a void in any heart, so wide and deep that nothing but the width and depth of vast eternity can fill it up!

Charles Dickens, *Dombey and Son*

CHAPTER 1

Good beginnings

Hugh J. Heggarty

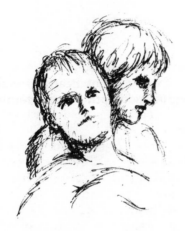

For 20 years or more as a consultant paediatrician in a general hospital I have had to pass on serious or very bad news to parents of children with newly discovered handicapping conditions or diseases which were likely to cause the death of the child either in the immediate future or in the next few months or years. What follows is a collection of memories, impressions, anecdotes, observations and comments in an attempt to share my stumbling, fumbling efforts and experiences with someone who may be in a similar and difficult situation now, or in the future. I do not myself have a handicapped child, nor have I ever experienced receiving news of permanent ill health in any of my children.

FIRST FEARS OF THE PARENTS – BREAKING BAD NEWS

All such situations vary enormously with the child, the nature of the problem, the family and the doctor. Only recently I had to explain to unsuspecting parents of a 22-month-old girl that she had a large abdominal mass which we quickly confirmed was a Wilm's tumour.

This sort of information, its timing and its unexpectedness, is not the same as when an obviously malformed baby is born.

Again this is unexpected, but in this situation the parents can see and already appreciate that there is something wrong.

Neither of these situations compares with the one in which parents first approach a family doctor with anxieties about their child's health and development. I am certain that all doctors who work with children should accept that the best observers of that child are his parents, particularly his mother, and we should take a very real interest when a mother is anxious about a 'falling off' in her child's progress or a loss of skills which he had previously possessed. In these circumstances it would not be sufficient to say that the development of this child was within the normal range if his parents are convinced that the child's skills are regressing. It is very rare in my experience for parents to take exception to a doctor's saying that he is not sure whether there is a serious problem. The important thing is that he should maintain interest and a willingness to share those concerns until the child's condition improves, a diagnosis is made, or a referral to a specialist centre becomes appropriate.

I have learned much from several doctors, such as Gerry Solomons and Ray Remboldt in Iowa City, USA, Trevor Wright at the Ryegate Centre for Children in Sheffield, Dick Ellis at the Child Development Centre in Newcastle upon Tyne and the late Ronnie McKeith in the Necoomen Centre, Guy's Hospital, London, as well as from chaplains and other medical and paramedical colleagues, but my most valuable lessons were from the children and their parents themselves. All of these experts with whom I have had the great privilege of working in the past agreed on the 'importance of the right start'. The initial interviewer is probably the most important person the family will meet and he sets the climate for the future. All of these doctors stressed to me the parents' need for adjustment, the precious gift of time, and repeated interviews. We need to check at regular intervals the stage which the parents have reached in their understanding, acceptance or despair. The parental reactions to 'bad news' no matter how sympathetically and gently broken, may be very varied indeed, whether the news is of a chronic condition (not necessarily life threatening) or of a life-threatening condition which may in fact result in the child's death within a few hours or days.

Some of the reactions I myself have encountered during such interviews will each be discussed in turn.

Biological

This tends to take two forms in my experience. The first is a desperate wish by loving parents to **protect** the helpless or the dying. This is, in itself, totally understandable from a human point of view and obviously must be encouraged. There is however, the danger of the affected child becoming almost a 'tyrant' in his own family. I believe that the presence in a family of a dying child, or the child with a life-long handicap, may in the very long term have a beneficial effect on that family. However, I would like to register my own protest against the idea that the presence of such children is always an unqualified blessing. Many times the parents, the siblings and close relatives and friends have commented to me how much their lives had been enriched by a child with a chronic or a fatal illness and I am well aware of the truth of that concept. Equally I have powerful and abiding memories of the 'tyranny' exerted by a particular handicapped child on the other members of his family and especially on his mother. So much attention was paid to the handicapped and seriously ill child that his 7-year-old sibling made a serious and almost successful attempt at suicide. I feel we have to qualify the excessively 'spiritual' attitude which is sometimes promoted by well-meaning and perhaps religiously motivated doctors, nurses and helpers. Not every handicapped child proves to be a 'blessing'.

Another biological reaction which I have witnessed is a feeling of **'revulsion at the abnormal'**, particularly in social classes 1 and 2 if there is more than a hint of mental retardation in the child, and particularly if there is a defect in the facial appearance of a newborn girl. A good example of the latter is cleft palate or any abnormality of the formation of the cranium. Many parents have told me that they could not bear to take the child out because she was female and had to live in a world where most people worship the big, the sexy and the beautiful ... a telling comment on today's values.

Inadequacy

Parents often express a feeling of inadequacy after the painful initial interview. Here both mother and father seem to feel that they have been inadequate in the basic act of human reproduction in so far as the child produced by them has a major defect or is going to die from disease. In addition, parents often fear inadequacy in their ability to rear and look after the child who has such disabilities. In our society it has been my impression that the mother feels this more keenly than the father and that the latter makes frequent 'escapes', for example, to work, the pub, the club etc.

Guilt

In this area too there is often an enormous feeling of guilt and a tendency for individual parents to blame 'the other side' or to blame 'themselves'. This particularly applies to the mother. This feeling of shame is often expressed openly by the parents, but in some families I have known it to be permanent, yet hidden and suppressed, only to become apparent many years later and even after the death of the child.

Bereavement

Parents in these sad circumstances frequently experience bereavement and all its stages, either rapidly passed through or sequentially over many weeks or months. Dr Marshall Klaus, working with unsophisticated families in Nicaragua, described beautifully the many varied processes of bonding between a child and his parents around the time of birth, and I have observed several times how my attempts to break bad news can seriously affect this bonding process. It is as though these parents have to reconcile themselves to the loss of the normal child they had assumed they would have, and indeed dreamed they would have. The idea of consumerism has now spread to the previously completely natural role of parenthood. I have come across in recent years an increasing number of parents who, when the 'bad news' is conveyed to them, at the time of the child's birth or soon after, adopt what I call the 'Supermarket' attitude and feel that their baby should 'be taken back' and replaced by a model without any faults! This is, of course, an over-simplification, but antenatal diagnosis, the idea that everyone is entitled to a perfect child and the suggestion in television drama programmes that doctors can 'fix everything' have led some families to believe that they are entitled to a normal child, that the odds are totally in their favour and that doctors should prevent abnormalities in 100% of cases. Such parents find it very difficult indeed to accept any defect in their offspring. Like a customer who has bought goods that are later found to be chipped, broken or faulty in some way, they demand to see the store manager and have an immediate replacement!

Shock

It is, of course, no surprise that another element of parental reaction is shock – a mixture of anger, disbelief and grief before any form of adjustment takes place. It is a perfectly natural tendency to blame someone, somehow, somewhere, for the news that their child has a major defect or a lethal disease. Some painful experiences over many years have taught me that one reaction of parents in such circumstances can be aggression. The bearer of bad news often becomes the target of the parent's anger. In perinatal events it is traditional to blame the family doctor, the obstetrician, the midwife, the anaesthetist or the attendant if the child is born with major problems and I myself have been physically assaulted on a few occasions by very angry mothers or fathers in the immediate aftermath of breaking the news, however gently it was done. It is said that in ancient Greece the bearer of bad news, for example a messenger who ran from the scene of a battle to his king to announce defeat, might well be executed! It is an important lesson for junior doctors and paramedical staff to understand that during the period of shock one of the basic human reactions may well be aggression directed at them, however innocent they may be.

Hope for a 'magic solution'

Often linked with denial by the parents is a tendency to 'go shopping for a magic solution'. Sadly, this sometimes takes parents on 'wild goosechases' to expensive units either in this country or elsewhere because such units may have a reputation in the popular press for magic cures or solutions to chronic handicap or lethal disease. This again is an all too natural and easily understood response by parents who are desperate. In such circumstances it is difficult for the doctor or nurse to be realistic without appearing to be cruel and heartless. I aim to reassure such parents that if a 'magic cure' for any of these conditions were available then the news would spread like wildfire around the medical centres of the world.

At times I feel that extravagant claims made by some doctors and their helpers in such centres do a great disservice to the patients and their parents in the long run. These comments are not meant to discourage genuine well-thought out trials of new therapies, but are an attempt to prevent parents building false hopes and becoming even more hurt.

I have no objection to 'alternative medicine' or homeopathic therapies, or using a 'healing ministry'. The only proviso in using these methods, alongside traditional medical ones, would be the maxim attributed to Florence Nightingale, 'First do no harm'.

Wish to be rid of 'the burden'

A possible reaction of parents is the wish to be rid of the burden. This feeling too is perfectly understandable either on a short-term or long-term basis and may well be a conscious or subconscious emotion. Occasionally I have seen it produce what I call 'the martyrdom complex' in which the parent or parents use the child as 'a cross' they must bear and with which they berate an apparently impotent and uncaring society.

Rejection

Rejection may have many aspects:

1. Rejection of the news.
2. Rejection of the help offered.
3. Rejection of the child by the parents.
4. Rejection of the child by the doctors and nurses because they feel that they have lost their role as curers of disease.

Some of these parents withdraw completely from society and reject the help offered by those who love them. The devastating news of a major malformation or a chronic life-threatening condition may provoke rejection which can in some instances be cold and calculated, in others totally irrational, in others still 'dutiful', in that the parent carries out the duties of parenthood without love. At times the rejection is theatrical and hysterical, but is none the less real to the parent. Rejection of the damaged or dying child can be immediate or sub-consciously life-long.

The rejecters need help, and doctors and nurses themselves have to recognize that there may well be occasions when they too are over-whelmed by the enormity of the problem to such an extent that they condone and cooperate with the rejection of the child.

Ray Remboldt taught me that doctors must realize that these feelings of parents are natural and normal and that they affect significantly the development and functioning of the child, however long or short that child's future may be. Dr Eric Denhoff, from Rhode Island, USA, stresses too that the attitude and cooperation of the parents are more important than the severity of the handicapping condition, even when the prognosis includes sadness and a short life. In the few studies on these topics in the USA I have noted that the father's views are almost always not mentioned. This is a major omission and may invalidate many claims made by authors on these topics. For ethical reasons too there have been very few experimental studies in methods of dealing with 'breaking the bad news'. The logistics of this are, of course, extremely difficult.

There seem to me to be class differences in UK families in the accept-ance of a retardate or a dying child; perhaps this is because of differing expectations. Indeed I suspect that the previous expectations held by parents before the child's birth are crucial. I have noted these class differences too in the attitudes of prospective adopters or foster parents and it interests me that amongst the rare 'parenting geniuses' whom I have met on a few occasions, there have been no such class-determined attitudes to overcome as they fall in love with the affected child.

The above classification of parental reactions is, of course, not wholly mine and is a composite made up from previous publications and from personal advice given to me by experts in this field. A much simpler classification of reactions devised by myself might have an appeal to the less academic spirits amongst us.

1. **'Emotionally shattered'** – usually painfully obvious, though not always.
2. **Defence mechanisms** – for example, many parents will say 'nobody told me anything' although someone may have tried for many hours and on many different occasions to transmit the bad news. Sometimes when parents say 'nobody told me anything' that is, in fact, sadly true but I would like to believe that paediatricians, nurses and social workers who work in this field, generally do their very best to communicate. We all, of course, have different skills in these areas and some are bound to do better than others.
3. **Mature adaptation** – there are many superb examples of wonderful families whose love for their children has overcome all the difficulties even if the end result was the untimely death of a much-loved child. For me the unexpected outcome is that in many such families both the child who is suffering and his parents and friends can provide a role model for others, enrich peoples lives and leave, in general, happy memories for their carers and their friends.

WHAT SHOULD THE DOCTOR SAY?

There are two interlinked aspects to this vexed question: What should the doctor say? and What are the parents' needs?

Convey accurate information honestly

In these difficult circumstances it is not always possible to do this in one session or even several split sessions. I spent over 11 hours in the home of a baby who had been diagnosed as having severe intracranial problems and cerebral palsy. These 11 hours were split up into seven or eight sessions and at the end of each of them I tried to 'recap' with the parents what had been said and tried to explore their understanding of the current situation. Yet when that family moved to another town and the parents were questioned by other doctors and paramedical staff about the information which had been given by me concerning their child the parents answered 'he did not tell me anything'. Either I am a desperately bad communicator or there is something which interferes with the reception of bad news. Perhaps in this case it was a mixture of both.

Interestingly enough, in an 'old fashioned' hospital which housed children and adults on a long-term basis because their families could not cope, I discussed this topic of 'breaking bad news' with the parents of perhaps 20 Down's syndrome adults and adolescents. Almost all of them complained that the news had been given to them in an unacceptable fashion and yet when I genuinely asked them for their own blue print as to how it should have been done, there were almost 20 individual versions offered. None the less, all of them stressed that it would be better to break bad news to both parents, and not to tell lies! I personally prefer to break bad news to both parents in their own home, if at all possible, and with grandparents around or even in the same room, if the parents so wish. The desperately difficult subject of what to tell the child himself, how, and when to involve him etc. is dealt with elsewhere in this book by writers more suited to this task than I am.

Allay anxiety and guilt

In such circumstances, to allay anxiety and guilt is very, very difficult, particularly if the defect is chromosomal or genetic or if one of the parents or close relatives has the same disease as the child himself. In these circumstances I have found it very helpful to call on the academic skills of the geneticists and the counselling skills of individual social workers, nurses and chaplains.

Eliminate the prejudices of the parents and society

I have mentioned already the tendency in today's world to emphasize the big, the beautiful, the wealthy and the sexy, and the true value of each individual child however handicapped, or however cruel may be the lethal disease from which he is suffering, tends to be submerged. I often ask myself where on this scale of human values in today's society do we find genuine love? I have to confess my own prejudices here. I feel quite strongly that abortion, infanticide, euthanasia and some aspects of ante-natal screening have not helped in this constant battle to afford to each individual person the importance and the dignity to which I believe he is entitled as a member of the human race. Professor Jerome Lejeune who, as a young scientist, discovered the chromosome abnormality in Down's syndrome and the Cri-du-Chat syndrome, in an oration to a medical society meeting in 1987 demanded in a plaintive fashion of an apparantly uncaring world, 'Man can go to the moon, why cannot he rear a Down's syndrome child? ... A feeble-minded fly is still a fly. ... When is a person?'

I believe that if doctors can 'de-personalize' a handicapped child in their own minds, then the way in which they present information to the parents will inevitably reflect that. In the 1970s the father of a newly born Down's syndrome child asked a paediatric colleague of mine to ensure that child's death by the intravenous injection of insulin. When my colleague protested that we were not in the business of killing babies, the child's father's reply was chilling: 'Last year over 200 000 babies were aborted in the United Kingdom. Only a tiny percentage of these were done because of physical abnormality, the rest could be described as inconvenient. I now order you to destroy my child who has medical difficulties and is far from normal.' There is a certain chilling logic in this statement. I have no doubt that attitudes towards the unborn potentially damaged child spill over into attitudes towards the born child who has disability, malformation or a lethal disease. In the 1980s the parents of a newborn spina bifida child suspected me of being one of those doctors 'who feed only dextrose and water to severely affected spina bifida neonates'. This was the first time in my medical career that I had been suspected by parents of doing ill to my patient. They misunderstood why 'clear fluids' (dextrose and water) had been given to this particular child, namely there was an anxiety that the child might have tracheo-oesophageal fistula in addition to her other difficulties and because milk down such a fistula could have caused serious lung problems, clear fluids were given as a precaution. Fortunately she did not have this defect and survived.

What can the child achieve and at what rate?

Sometimes the doctor has to admit honestly that this is guesswork. My senior colleagues in the field of handicap warned me that it is sometimes a mistake to give too much information all at once and too quickly, and that the news is best given gradually and repeated at short intervals. I do not think this can be applied to families whose children are likely to die of a serious metabolic defect or neoplastic disease in the fairly near future. In such circumstances information has to be given promptly, no matter how painful that may be to all concerned.

Set goals of management

In some children, for example, there may be a temporary improvement in a physical disability. We should always strive to provide enjoyable and interesting educational opportunities for such children and foster desirable personality development, even if the future is determined in terms of days or weeks. The parents are the key and should be encouraged to concentrate on day-to-day matters as much as possible; this is again something that other contributors to this book can more usefully address (see especially Chapter 4).

Will it happen again?

Parents are entitled to a clear answer to this question, if indeed a straightforward answer is readily available to the doctor. If not, then the doctor must obtain this information via his nearest genetic service (usually based in a university teaching hospital). I have seen serious repercussions from failure to do this, for example, parents who have not been informed that they are carriers of a lethal or serious medical condition producing more children without the prior information to which they have a basic right. It is the informant's duty to pass on the facts. The parents then may have difficult decisions to make, but the least they deserve is adequate information, correctly timed.

The six major aspects discussed above have a very important impact on the relationships between the doctor who is breaking the bad news and the family who are receiving it. It is crucial that other medical and paramedical agencies close to the family are appropriately informed, clearly, and at the same time or within a day or two. On this point the family doctor is central to the support for the family, especially when the consultant may be in a specialist unit some distance from the child's home. It is important that he is given accurate information promptly about the child's condition, the likely progression of the disease and the future medical management, if any. I believe that it is especially important that the staff in the specialist unit stress and enhance the family doctor's role. A phone call between the two doctors is by far the best method and it is equally important that any therapists, nurses and 'alternative practitioners' are given satisfactory and adequate explanation of the child's problems by the specialist concerned. Without this communication there is much room for confusion and unlimited scope for further pain to be inflicted unwittingly on the child and his family.

PITFALLS

There are many pitfalls to be avoided – some are mistakes that I have made myself, and I suspect others have made them too.

'Over-diagnosis'

Over-diagnosis can sometimes confuse rather than help. The simpler the statement the better, although some of today's metabolic diseases confuse even the best brains and attempting to explain, say, mucopolysaccharidosis to distraught parents is not easy. I find that the initial transfer of news in such circumstances may be quite brief, but that I set up a meeting with both parents and/or anyone else they may wish to nominate to come along, for example relatives, chaplain etc., as soon as possible on their own territory and on their own terms. This has proved very useful on many occasions.

Paralysis

The public have the image of the doctor as a 'cure all'; on television he is usually an heroic figure. The excitement of fictional and real life medical programmes can often exaggerate amongst laymen the skill of doctors, and the fact that the child may have an incurable disease can often induce a feeling of paralysis in the parents and in the doctors. The blow to their ego can be devastating. It is important for doctors in such circumstances to recognize that they perhaps are not the best persons to be attempting to pass on bad news if they know that they themselves have major difficulties in accepting any kind of failure.

Doctors' anger if the diagnosis is questioned

It is sometimes very difficult for parents in these awkward consultations to question the correctness of the doctor's diagnosis. Some senior doctors feel greatly threatened, and indeed angry, if a layman questions their medical diagnosis. This is regrettable, and should be avoidable, provided both parties are honest and gentle in their approach.

In general I try to dissuade parents from 'shopping' round other centres in desperation, although it is very hard to persuade them not to. I myself am very ready to offer a second medical opinion if I feel it is in the best interests of the child or the parents, or even if I feel there is little likelihood of a different opinion from the one sadly given by myself. In some cases I would encourage the parents to have at least one further opinion. This is usually because there is a major anxiety for such parents in accepting my opinion, and I have no compunction in recommending an expert to see them. Fortunately the medical profession has many brave, conscientious and knowledgeable experts in the field of rare diseases in childhood and I am pleased to acknowledge here the tremendous help I have been given by paediatric colleagues with specialist knowledge. I am always reassured when such doctors with brilliant minds also turn out to have gentle and caring hearts.

Failure to listen

Just listening to parents is often a form of therapy. I am guilty of talking too much. One of my close friends once asked me 'Have you ever wondered why God gave you two ears and one mouth?' My medical training prepared me poorly or not at all for these very difficult personal situations in which the doctor has to learn to listen as well as to take the lead in conversations. Dr Trevor Wright of Sheffield gave parents much comfort from the apparently simple and patient manner of his attentiveness and listening skills. His watching, gentle presence carried as much influence with anxious parents as his occasional moments of professional advice or replies to specific questions and in this area he epitomized a model which every good doctor should try to emulate.

Failure to allow parents to ventilate their feelings

This has been touched on earlier. Aggression and anger may have to be ventilated there and then or at some time in the future. It is useful, I think, to lead the parents towards a diagnosis and to a 'consensus conversation' with their friends, relatives, the medical adviser and the chaplain.

Rejection

Rejection of the bad news may not just be felt by parents. The diagnosis and prognosis may in some rare instances be rejected, consciously or subconsciously, by grandparents, siblings, doctors and nurses too. I think a domiciliary visit here is very important and should be more often used. It is useful for the medical adviser to tackle 'head on' some of the objections and denials of relatives who love the child so much that they cannot bear to admit the presence of a dread disease. These objections and denials of the child's problems can greatly inhibit the adaptation which is necessary for mature acceptance.

Always leave hope

Although we should not raise false hopes about the possible length of life, we can usually give hope for the quality of life that remains. We can reassure the family that we are not abandoning the child, and will provide active palliative care. The time that the family have left with the child is especially precious because it is short. Their love is the most important thing to offer the child.

Do not over-doctor

Although it is important that families do not feel abandoned by their hospital doctor, other professionals often have a far more important role to play than he has. These include the family doctor, health visitor, social worker, therapists and child development centre and other non-medical staff. Parent support groups are often a source of great strength.

It is important to tell parents about support groups as early as possible. How soon families contact these groups varies from family to family. I think the ideal is to pass the information on clearly to the family and leave them in control. Sometimes the availability of the name and address coupled with the willingness of that doctor or that group to be available is all that the family requires.

FACTORS THAT HELP

Some factors that I think help in this situation are:

1. Use a child-centred approach.
2. Treat parents as the key team members.
3. Employ patience and persistence.
4. Use group experiences.
5. Recognize a plateau of achievement.
6. Educate the professionals.

The list is not comprehensive; I have no doubt my colleagues could supply many more.

Child-centred approach

It is essential to concentrate on the child rather than the disease or the handicap from which the child suffers. The doctor should hold the baby or child during the interview or, at least, sit down near to the child and the parents so that there is some sense of physical contact. I have had no training whatsoever in the psychology of 'body language' etc., but I feel this is a natural human reaction and that it is far better if the doctor feels part of a group rather than someone dispensing wisdom from 'on high' in a detached fashion. I remember distantly in my medical training being told that it is a bad thing for doctors to become emotionally involved with their patients. I can understand the wisdom of that advice, but it is a sweeping statement and when it applies to a paediatrician and the family facing desperately bad news I think it is totally impractical. It is my own view that to be totally neutral in such circumstances is neither possible nor desirable.

Parents are the key members of the team

Whether it is a child development centre or a hospice which is planning the management of a dying child, the parents are the key members of the team. Doctors should treat them as such. I find it helpful sometimes to advise such parents to try to forget the weeks and months that perhaps stretch before them and to concentrate rather on the day which is definitely coming tomorrow. 'In the dark, do not look at the horizon, look at your feet.'

Patience and persistence are crucial

Criticism and impatience are destructive elements in any child's life. They are absolutely lethal to the spirit of a handicapped or dying child.

Group experiences can be very valuable

In general I would be opposed to the 'shutting away' response of some parents. I fully understand that a close-knit family will perhaps wish to manage privately its own individual grief and bereavement reactions at the time of the child's death and thereafter. None the less, there can be very valuable support from groups such as might exist in a village, a school, a church or a religious community. I personally feel, in such a circumstance, when I visit the home of a dying child or one who has died recently, that the role of the doctor has been described beautifully by Harvey Markovitch, when he referred to meetings with groups of parents for other reasons – 'The doctor should shut up and listen'.

The plateau of achievement

If a plateau of achievement is reached in a handicapped child's development, it is best to say so and help the parents accept the child's maximal capacities at that time. The same applies to a child who is dying, for example a child with cystic fibrosis or a progressive cancer. There does come a time, which Janet Goodall describes so clearly and empathically in her chapter (Chapter 2) when major attempts to prolong the child's life are withdrawn and the focus thereafter is to enhance the quality and the value of the life that remains.

Educate the professionals

This applies to doctors, health visitors, social workers, teachers and all whose professional role brings them in contact with a severely handicapped or dying child. Medical students need to learn about the special needs of the dying or the handicapped; I cannot recall this ever being discussed during my own six years of undergraduate training. Child development centres, district handicap teams, family support units and residential social services establishments are sometimes very helpful as training centres for many disciplines. I believe that a specialist team may well be required in each district to try to override the boundaries between various departments in this sensitive area of chronic handicap and/or the dying child. It is my opinion that doctors themselves suffer from the handicap of a tradition of elevated status and superior knowledge. A great barrier to provision of proper follow-up services and care is the clumsy and divisive nature of the health service organizations, particularly the unfortunate split between community and hospital facilities for children. I am delighted that the British Paediatric Association and the Faculty of Community Medicine recognize that this split is not to the advantage of healthy children and certainly works to the great disadvantage of the families of children with lethal disorders.

I stress again that breaking bad news will never be an easy task. There are no blueprints, no code of practice to guide us on how to break bad news to the parents of a child with a major handicapping or lethal condition. None the less, we could be guided by the following quotations – 'Nature has given man the power to weep, perhaps that is the best part of us' (Juvenal); 'People more than things need to be restored, reclaimed, revived, redeemed, redeemed and redeemed – never throw out anybody' (Levison); and finally a beautiful quotation from the nurse of a dying child – 'Perhaps the poet better than the physician feels the pulse of mankind.'

FURTHER READING

Chapman, Jennifer and Goodall, Janet (1979) Dying children need help too. *British Medical Journal*, 1, 593–4.
Cunningham, C.C., Morgan, P.A. and McGucklen, R.B. (1984) Down syndrome – is dissatisfaction with disclosure of the diagnosis inevitable? *Developmental Medicine and Child Neurology*, 26, 33–9.
Klaus, Marshall and Fararoff, A.A. (1986) Care of the parents, in *Care of the High Risk Neonate*, Saunders, Philadelphia, ch. 7, pp. 147–70.
McKeith, Ronald C. (1963) The care of mentally subnormal children. *Developmental Medicine and Child Neurology*, 5(6), 557–8.
Rembolt, Raymond (1960) *Talking to Parents*, University of Iowa, Iowa City.
Saunders, Cicely (1978) *The Management of Terminal Disease*, Arnold, London.
Solomons, Gerald (1965) What do you tell the parents of a retarded child? *Clinical Paediatrics*, 4(4).
Solomons, Gerald and Menolascino, Frank (1968) Importance of a right start. *Clinical Paediatrics*, 7(1).

CHAPTER 2

Thinking like a child about death and dying

Janet Goodall

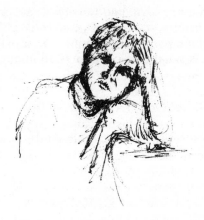

One of the worst things about most adults is that they have forgotten what it was like to be a child. Serious failures of communication can occur when important information is offered to children by those who are unaware of the need for different age groups to be approached differently. Children are not all attuned to the same wavelength, and what seems straightforward to an older mind can have quite a different connotation for a young one. The writer Laurie Lee (of *Cider with Rosie* fame) tells us how on his first day at primary school he was allocated a place in the classroom and told to 'sit there for the present'. At the end of the day he went home disappointed and upset because he had never been given his present. Such understandable confusion added to his trauma on leaving the security of home for the first time. Amusing as such stories are to adult minds, they are serious and upsetting misconceptions for a child.

How much more distressed children may be when someone dear to them is very ill or dying but explanations are either not broached at all, or are in such veiled terms as to be meaningless or mystifying. Confidence can be shaken for ever if what is believed to have been said by a hitherto trusted adult turns out not to be the case, so, in the child's mind, it is all a lie. Lies can be real as well as imagined. When a pet dies, it is not unusual for parents to rush out to replace it, pretending that the old one got lost, or even trying to pass off the new budgie as still being the old one. It would be better to let this be a learning experience by helping the child to face and accept the truth. Those of us who face with parents a death in the family, perhaps hardest of all the death of their child, may have to interpret for them remarks or questions which can come from young relatives and friends as well as from a dying child. Parents are not necessarily experts in understanding children and are often grateful to be helped with this, but caregivers themselves may also have to relearn the language of childhood, which is what this chapter is all about.

THINKING LIKE A CHILD

It is only in this century that progress has been made in describing the conceptual growth of young children by pioneers such as Jean Piaget, whose observations on his own children formed a basis for further study and analysis by others. Babies at birth have now been so closely observed that we have a clearer idea than ever before of the way that the growing mind normally develops, from the neonatal period right up to adolescence and so into adulthood [1]. At each stage, babies, infants, children and young people can all have additional problems if those caring for them overlook, in their management, the child's need for understanding and comprehensive explanation.

EARLY MONTHS

It was perhaps the hospitalization of birth that first impeded, but then invited, the recognition that personal relationships are important to babies as well as to their parents. Child abuse was found to be much more likely in children who had been separated at birth from their parents [2]. Babies have an innate readiness to attune to sensory input of all kinds [3], of which parents can be quite ignorant [4] but which, if encouraged, enhances the growth of good relationships. By 6 weeks a baby can indicate recognition of a familiar face and by 5 months gives a delighted welcome back to a special person who has been temporarily absent. Although out of sight to the infant means out of existence until about 10 months of age, the development of a concept of permanence then means that unseen objects and people are now realized still to exist even when they have disappeared from view.

Setting this in the context of our discussion, this means that a dying baby or infant is not too small to value and to need contact, not merely with professional caregivers but most particularly with someone who is emotionally close. Comfort may best be found in familiar arms as much as (though often as well as) through analgesia.

Follow-up was arranged with 44 couples whose baby, born with spina bifida but unsuitable for surgery, had died (when more than a week old) during 1971–81, up to 15 years before the interviews. Between 1971 and 1976 no such baby had ever gone home, but by 1981, 92 per cent of such children were receiving palliative and often terminal care at home. The difference in the resolution of their parents' grief varied strikingly with the degree of involvement which they had been encouraged to have with their child. More than a decade later many of those who had felt excluded by the hospital remained angry and bitter that, as they felt, their baby had experienced such a rotten life. Those who had cared for their own baby had a much sweeter sadness, esteeming the child to have had a life made as good as was possible because of their own personal care [5].

The bad old practice of excluding parents from neonatal and any other units has finally been recognized and corrected at most major centres, though this can still cause problems when a specialist centre is away from the home base. That the parents' presence matters to an infant may influence a decision to allow a baby (for example, with inoperable congenital heart disease) to return home for palliative and terminal care, or alternatively to help parents to be there to discuss the switching off of a no longer useful ventilator. It is sobering to think how recently it is that these practices have come into force, to help both the patient, the parents and, more recently still, other siblings.

In many parts of the world, sick children are still treated as hospital property, particularly where the possibility of palliative care is still a new idea, with an accordingly poor life for the child and pathological grief for the family.

FROM 1 TO 3 YEARS OLD

By their first birthday most children can, with help, stand up and look around. For the first time they can now connect their previous view of the four legs of a chair or table with its upper surface. The whole perspective is changed.

What previously could be hurled out of sight and so out of mind is now seen still to be there. Yet there are more connections to be made.

It is all right to throw balls but not bread. It is acceptable to put a sticky mug on to the kitchen table but not on to the piano. This is increasingly the age range for copying what adults do, but, as at this stage two ideas only can be matched at once, some vital component may be left out. Pouring milk into the cereal packet shows a recognition of two major ingredients for the usual nice breakfast, but by leaving out other important stages in the process a child may be dismayed to arouse a domestic storm instead of being congratulated for achievement. Trying to toast a piece of paper instead of a piece of bread can cause a conflagration and inedible mess, the different degrees of flammability and edibility being unknown to a young mind. The legacy of a residual guilt imposed by such disasters will depend on the general level of warmth and understanding in that home.

Parental tension can mount as the state known as negativism emerges. It is common to most children in this age group but alarming to novices whose docile, smiling infant suddenly becomes expert at emptying cupboards, shredding important papers, and anointing furniture with toothpaste (or worse) or simply saying an immovable 'No'. This is all normal, giving evidence of emerging independence, but it not only alarms the parents; it can actually be very frightening to a young child to discover so much power unless protected by the establishment of clear limits. A parental attitude of firm, affectionate expectancy, that these lessons will slowly be learned and observed, gives great security. It has to be remembered, the egocentricity is not the deliberately self-centred adult version of this stage but an outlook which genuinely cannot be helped except by time and teaching. It takes years for a child to be able to think in any depth from someone else's viewpoint. Even though a 2-year-old seeing a mother's tears may say, 'Don't cry, Mummy', this is likely to be copying what the mother has often said herself rather than entering into the reason for the tears, though there is probably also an element of affectionate concern for someone near and dear being so sad. Teaching social skills and concern can be a long hard struggle and it is not easy being either parent or child while this is going on. Overzealous discipline can leave a legacy of guilt, but lack of control is equally disastrous; getting the balance right is a learning process for all [6]. The way in which parents have handled family discipline is likely to influence the way that their child copes with the rigours of a life-threatening illness.

Unless parents are accustomed to offering anticipatory explanations to a child, a hospital admission, with its attendant personal discomforts and inconveniences, may be perceived by the child as punishment or, if left for long hours alone in a strange cot, as rejection. Yet even the normal state of negativism can mean that a spoonful of medicine provokes a furore. Parents can be embarrassed, but also pleasantly surprised, by their child's responses to new stresses.

best if they themselves have been briefed as to what is going ,appen so that they can forewarn the child in their own familiar way, but this means that the professional team must first take time to explain it to them, possibly with suggestions to less confident parents as to how to express the information. Time spent in this way is more likely to win the child's cooperation and so is well invested. It can also reassure nervous parents who might otherwise have been inclined to leave the child to get on without them. It is better for them to warn that something will hurt just a little but be over quickly than to say that it will not hurt. 'You may want to cry, but I'll hold you' can be more reassuring than giving orders not to cry at all. A strongly supported child makes professional tasks so much easier.

The major consolation for parents of children under 3 years old who are dying will be that they are unaware of their own serious state and their egocentric minds will not look ahead and ask awkward questions. 'Why?' questions come later: this age group is more likely to make 'I' statements, such as 'I don't want it, I don't like it'. Here, imagination can help, but dithering will only hinder. Thus, an iced lolly or ice-chip will freeze the taste buds before unpalatable drugs need to be taken, but that they have to be taken is then part of the deal. Three-year-olds are particularly responsive to appeals to their being so much bigger and more helpful than anyone smaller would be, a remark worth slipping in early on in a procedure, in a matter-of-fact rather than pleading manner, to produce maximum effect.

Parents are more likely to worry about how to help brothers and sisters in this age group who have a dying sibling. The answer is to let them be involved, even to the point of letting them see the baby after death. This is likely to be such an appalling idea to many parents that it may have to be gently broached ahead of time. No child should be forced into this situation, any more than adults should decisively exclude children from it. Yet there is likely to be great anxiety about a beloved brother who has mysteriously disappeared; 'Is it because I hit him?' may never be said out loud. Being taken to see him, even when he eventually seems very quiet and still, can be a help in facing the reality which no amount of words could explain to such an inexperienced mind.

Clearly, terminal care in the home is a better option if this can be managed as encounters will happen more naturally both before and after death. Even a 2-year-old can recognize a dead butterfly, bird or pet by its immobility and lack of response when touched, but the finality of death is not comprehended at this age. Adult fears of such an encounter being upsetting reflect their own perceptions rather than those of a very young child. Understandably, it is distressing to adults to contemplate letting this happen, but in retrospect they may find that it is actually strangely comforting to them as well as being of value to their children.

An infant of 10 months old was admitted to an intensive care unit with an acute respiratory illness, her mother staying at the hospital to be near her. The 3-year-old sister was very anxious at their disappearance overnight and intensive care unit staff were prevailed upon to invite her to come and see what was going on. They had some evident trepidation, as the infant had an indwelling naso-endotracheal tube which they thought would be frightening. There was, therefore, an air of 'I told you so' when the child arrived and stood at the door of the unit within sight of her mother, but refused at first to go in further.

Fortunately, this was recognized as being a signal to her mother of her need for reassurance that both children were still in favour, and that she had not deliberately chosen to leave home taking the little one with her. With encouragement, the child went in and sat on her little sister's bed with only a dismissive glance at her new proboscis. There was an immediate improvement in the patient's level of interest as well as relief of the sister's own anxiety. Her major query then was why had she been told that her mother had gone to sleep with Laura, when she was in such a little cot that this was clearly untrue. Inspection of the nearby Z-bed melted that suspicion and all went well from then on with both children.

A 7-year-old died suddenly of cystic fibrosis, also on an intensive care unit. Her 2-year-old sister was brought in to see what had happened and to kiss her goodbye. This she did quite calmly, saying 'Goodnight' and using her sister's name. That she still asked when her sister would be coming home did not diminish the importance of this little ceremony. It indicated her lack of understanding about death's irreversibility rather than the belief that her sister had simply gone to sleep, despite her normally laboured breathing having stopped.

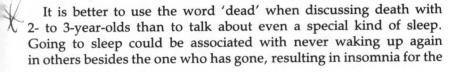

It is better to use the word 'dead' when discussing death with 2- to 3-year-olds than to talk about even a special kind of sleep. Going to sleep could be associated with never waking up again in others besides the one who has gone, resulting in insomnia for the

3-year-old and repeated nocturnal visits to wake up parents, possibly for weeks to come.

FROM 3 TO 6 YEARS OLD

Matching one thing to another becomes increasingly skilful across this age span, smaller and smaller categories being compared and contrasted. Not only can harder jigsaws be tackled but the hierarchies within a hospital team are slowly sorted out. Insight, however, is still largely lacking and although adult phraseology and explanation may be confidently repeated this can be rote learning rather than true understanding. What is overheard from the bottom of the bed can be particularly likely to set off new fantasies, so that a personal explanation to the child, using drawings or puppets if need be, is a matter to be constantly recollected. One 5-year-old became unexpectedly withdrawn and worried after thinking that the doctor had said that he was going to get his 'deathoscope'. Fortunately his mother was quick to expose the error, with instant improvement in his demeanour and a speedier recovery.

It is wise to give a child the name of a life-threatening illness early on in its course as, although the full implications will not yet be grasped, it becomes a familiar term. As time goes on its portent will, of course, be realized so that updating information is an essential part of care. Unless a child is exceptionally bright, or experienced, penetrating questions or revised explanations are not likely to arise until about 6 years of age. Yet the exceptions must always be borne in mind and parents, as well as junior staff who are often closest to the patient, should be primed as to how to be most helpful when such needs arise.

More mysterious, and so worrying to the child, is when a word or activity which already has one use is applied differently (as with Laurie Lee and his 'present'). The manipulations performed by a physiotherapist can be puzzling if a child's similar handling of the baby had recently precipitated a domestic incident. Being told that tapping the chest is to make a cough go away is even more baffling if it seems that it at once has made it worse. An analogy with patting sauce out of the ketchup bottle may help, as the child can see that it has helped to bring up the sticky stuff which was so irritatingly tickly and so get the idea that the interventions are purposeful, not punitive.

The age of fantasy has clearly arrived for this age group, aided by television and the horror videos which so many families now watch. Dreams and nightmares can be thought of as real events. A significant percentage of 6-year-olds still think of death not only as reversible but as violent and horrible. Other children, on a ward or in a clinic, tell gruesome stories of how one of them may disappear without either reappearance of explanation. Children can believe the worst but ask no questions, believing their fears to be known and probably shared even by adults. It may only be by behavioural changes, such as lack of co-operation over clinic visits or therapy, or by insomnia, weepiness or enuresis, that the resultant anxiety state is suspected. Clues may be found in drawings or in play activities and become conversation openers, which will probably be more productive than would be more direct questioning about what is wrong.

Whether explaining an illness and its therapy or trying to interpret a child's anxieties, it is always helpful to imagine oneself back into the skin of a child of that age and to try to look at what is going on from a child's-eye viewpoint. The important thing to recall is that a young child tends to look at things with entirely superficial judgement, based on and matched with what has already been experienced. Events and their causes are commonly attributed to the self as either victim or responsible agent.

Add to this that his private thoughts are not recognized by the child as being private to him, and he therefore does not see the need to tell someone else about them. It is not surprising therefore that mismanagement of any kind of trauma at this stage of life and failure to help the child to comprehend it can have long-lasting repercussions into later life. In this context it will be of on-going importance to bereft children that their needs are understood. The dying child, too, may need help in sorting out fantasy from fact if there is to be peace of mind as the end approaches. A watchful eye and a sympathetic, attuned ear are as essential to the care of the dying child as are most of our drugs. Truth expressed in terms appropriate for the age will bring greater confidence and calm than would fobbing off a child. There is quick awareness of secrets, as well as great determination to fathom them, and an inbuilt need for trust.

A 5-year-old, very experienced after more than three years of cancer therapy, developed paraplegia and became blind in one eye. His friend had died of leukaemia. He asked his mother, out of the blue, 'Is it going to happen to me like it happened to David?' Her first shocked reaction was to say, 'Don't be so silly, of course not', and then to wish for the ground to swallow her up. Later he asked her directly, 'Am I going to die?' and this time she had courage to say 'Yes, we're all going to die and because you are so poorly, it looks as if you are going to die first, but it won't be today and we'll be with you.' At 5 years old he could match his own state to his old friend's and so expect the same outcome, but he did not yet have a mind mature enough to range very far ahead. His mother's answer satisfied him without his then feeling the need to ask, 'When will it be?' Not long afterwards he died quietly, still at home, with his parents present.

His sisters, aged 4 and 10 years old, had seen that he was not getting better. They had moved house a great deal, so when deterioration was advancing, their parents explained that Marc's body was like a house that was falling down and one day he would move out and leave it behind. When this eventually happened, their father brought them home from school and they chose to sit with their brother's body, letting the fact sink in that he had really gone. The older one commented later, without distress, that he had seemed 'peaceful, but different' [7].

When there is time, under 6-year-olds should be forewarned of an impending death in the family and any anticipatory fantasies earthed by the assurance that to die need not be very uncomfortable or lonely. All that young minds may need to know is that dear and special people will be there as company for the dying one. The idea of death as being the end of a person is not one that comes naturally to young children; older minds will grapple with questions about the after-life whereas little ones cannot conceive of anything else than of going on and on pretty much as before. This can pose problems for agnostic parents as to what they should say both to the dying child, and then to bereft siblings, but it is better to be honest with children than to produce explanations with a hollow ring which they all too quickly detect and suspect. For an unbelieving family to drag in God and his heaven at this stage is more likely to produce antipathy than relief, or a constant watchfulness of the skies while trying to spot the aeroplane which is carrying the dear departed. If, however, there is genuine faith and trust that the one who has gone has been received into the company of other names held dear, that can be the most comforting concept of all. Sometimes the trust of a very small child can turn doubting parents to faith.

A few days before being killed in a road accident, a small boy had asked his mother if Jesus would look after him when he went to sleep. To humour him, more than out of a great conviction, she had said that this would always be so. This was later recalled and provided faith and comfort to both parents as a belief to hold on to and a firm anchorage in the emotional upheaval which followed his sudden death.

FROM 6 TO 10 YEARS OLD

This is the age of making deductions, for putting two and two together with a fair chance of getting it right, although face value judgement can still come to the fore for any of us when facing new experiences and is particularly likely to mislead a slow or much protected child. Painful experiences are especially likely to accelerate growth, so that classification of conceptual development according to chronological age is only approximate. Children who have endured much during a chronic disability are likely to be ahead of their peers in understanding, hence the overlap in the subdivisions of age categorized in this discussion.

One way to assess how a child is likely to be looking at things is to offer a simple test which can be presented as a game. Six little men are put into six toy trucks, or some comparable arrangement, and the men then spread out into a longer row. The average 6-year-old is now likely to say that there are more men than trucks, even having seen the change being made. The next stage of the development is to recognize that there must still be the same number as they were the same at the start, this giving evidence of ability to make deductive reasoning. False deductions are not unusual though, and can give rise to unwarranted assumptions. Thus, an 8-year-old had already died of a disease which her younger sister knew that she also had, so on her own eighth birthday asked if she would now die, too. Fortunately she had a good enough relationship with her mother to ask and so to be truthfully reassured. Other such children may worry in silence.

Changes in behaviour at this age, such as lack of compliance with therapy, may be clues to the child's new way of looking at things. Drugs that may have been taken faithfully over years, such as for cystic fibrosis, may suddenly be questioned or refused, it now being easily deduced that other children are not required to take them. Therapy now needs to be explained in a new way. By 7 years old, simple diagrams can help a child to understand, for example, what effect bronchodilators have on the size of the tubes taking air to the lungs. Using imagery with which the child is familiar, such as comparing the bronchi to different sized straws or inflating the lungs to blowing up balloons, and likening the lung to an upside down tree in winter all helps to give a picture of what is going on to a mind which, despite fantasizing, had not previously been able to engage in imagining what goes on inside the body. The prevalence of computer war games will make it relatively easy to describe cytotoxic therapy as a secret agent put into the bloodstream to 'zapp' the enemy cells that are threatening to take over. There is still little insight, though, as to what the future may hold, with the notable exception, again, of a bright or greatly experienced child.

A boy with cystic fibrosis had been treated with physiotherapy, a special diet and intermittent antibiotics for most of his life, but at 6 years old he asked why his two brothers were not expected to have all this. Prior to this he had neither noticed nor been troubled about being different. Two years later he had a hospital admission, was very ill and then slow to recover. He suddenly asked his mother whether cystic fibrosis could kill. Very sensibly, she clarified first why he was asking this, realizing how easy it can be for an adult to give a child an answer to a question which is not the one that the questioner really had in mind. The boy exemplified this by then saying that he was afraid that when he died he would be cold and hungry down there by himself in the hole that dead people are put into. His mother reassured him that it would just be his body that was in the hole, like an old overcoat that he had finished with. He himself would be with Grandpa, who had recently died. They discussed this for almost two hours in a rare and deep conversation, after which he made a rapid physical improvement.

A life-threatening illness may go on for years, so it is important to remember that information which was given and accepted very simply at the start will need to be updated as time goes on. The patient's understanding about the illness and its therapy needs to grow with the child if both rebellion and confusion are to be averted. This is true, too, for other children in the family or school who are growing up under the same shadow.

A baby with spina bifida would not have been helped by surgery but went home without operation to live his short life with his family. His 6-year-old sister was thrilled to have him home, but when he was 6 weeks old on a follow-up hospital visit, the parents reported that she had 'gone off' the baby and now spent a lot of time playing outside. It was then realized that she had been told nothing about his disability, the parents not knowing what to say, but had clearly picked up something of their sadness and tried to distance herself from its cause. After discussion, they decided to tell her the truth, comforted her tears and welcomed her back into the close-knit foursome again. Supported, she could cope with reality far better than when worrying herself about an unshared secret.

FROM 10 YEARS TO ADOLESCENCE

This age group has no trouble at all with the man-and-lorry test. More complicated judgements can now be made, as shown by other simple exercises. If one of two equally filled and identical glasses were to be emptied into a tall cylindrical container in front of a group of children of different ages, their responses would show a maturation of concepts with their advancing ages. Up to 5 and 6 years old a child would be likely to say that there was more water in the cylinder than in the remaining glass. A child who had grasped the concept of reversibility would deduce that, whatever it all looked like, the volumes of water must be the same. Children over 10 years old would, with increasing confidence, be able to gauge volumes by eye, whether or not they had seen the transformation taking place. Ability to think in three dimensions has now arrived. With this would also come the ability to perceive that an illness is taking a downhill course and both patient and peers may slowly realize that death may not be far away. A change from active to palliative care is likely to be seen for what it is, so should not be made without discussion. Deductions may be correct, but imagination, while rich, is still uninformed. By now there will probably have been more visual input, with the possible viewing of scenes showing fearsome and unforgettable modes of death. Inner fears may need to be expressed, but are added to by fearing their confirmation. A gentle opener of conversation can bring relief, such as, 'Sometimes, when people are ill, they begin to wonder what will happen to them next'. The young person may or may not respond, but if the hint is taken up it is good to let the exchange then be paced by the patient. Truth is often more acceptable in stages.

For the sick child at the lower end of the age range and for the majority of well but concerned siblings and friends, parents or friendly adults are more likely to be chosen as confidants. As time goes on, questions and deeper conversations may more naturally arise with someone nearer in age, particularly with another teenager. The youngest paramedical on duty may thus be landed with a devastating question. To answer, 'I wonder what makes you ask me that just now?' gives a moment to regain poise, as well as ensuring that the question has really been understood. Anyone then feeling unable to cope further should at this point offer to find someone more skilled, rather than telling a transparent untruth or scuttling away on a suddenly recollected urgent task elsewhere. The one called upon to help may find that the question has already gone into cold storage, but is thereby primed to be ready another time. A low key conversation about sleep and dreams may bring into the discussion some of the fears and concerns which might have disturbed them. Artistic efforts by children of all ages may give windows into their minds as well as giving emotional release, when inner fantasies are externalized.

Parents may wish to put an embargo on any talk about prognosis with their dying child. The older child may not want anything of what has been said to be relayed back to the parents. Confidentiality towards both parties has to be respected, but honest sharing rather than subterfuge is the goal. Sometimes, new and perplexing symptoms arise which are entirely due to unresolved emotional or spiritual tension. Young children are likely to be mirroring their parents' anxiety, but even a reflective 10-year-old can have insight into the personal implications of continuing deterioration. Adolescents normally experience frequent mood swings, but these can be compounded by the classical components of grief and lost expectations [8]. Denial, anger and guilt (which is anger against oneself) depression and bargaining may all show up in different ways. Denial can bring a false facade of not caring, or can provoke an attempt at suicide. Anger, as in healthy adolescence, can be explosive and hard to deal with.

Guilt arises from seeing the sadness in others provoked by the continued illness. Depression deepens as old pursuits and some old friends fall away and suicidal feelings may recur. Siblings in this age group are likely to have similar feelings but show them in different ways, denial sometimes keeping them from visiting the one who is dying. Other emotions can result in behavioural disturbances, often completely out of character. Parents may be so caught up in their own feelings, and professionals so busy with the patient, that these very important needs may not be perceived. If not helped at this stage, or if death is sudden, they will surface strongly at the time of bereavement.

A 12-year-old girl died suddenly of a cerebral haemorrhage. Her teenage brother started to stay out late at night and became very rude and angry when his parents protested. They complained bitterly about his 'thoughtless behaviour at a time like this' without recognizing the signs of his own shock and sadness. The fact that his sister's death had come without warning left him unprepared and without any already involved professional there to help. When there is time to offer support during a long illness, the needs of more than patient and parents must be remembered.

Despite all the trauma and genuine anguish experienced by all involved in their care, as well as by dying young people themselves, many adolescents can be very impressive as they come through to the point of making the best of what life remains. This is usually the result of much personal care and support as well as, for some, the development of a personal faith in God. Trying to inflict unwanted conversation is, of course, to be avoided, but to find someone who is willing to open up on a hitherto taboo subject must be an immense relief. Feeling free to express so many pent up emotions, without any false reassurances or attempts to change the subject, and to find a sympathetic sharing in the sadness of decline, can actually bring about a surprising upturn in spirit and an improved sense of well-being. Achieving such a sense of trust often takes time and can take its own toll from the supporter, but is worth it all, especially if it leads to a greater openness within the family.

A young teenager had a leg amputated for osteosarcoma though she was told that it had been for infection. When a friend asked her what it was like to have cancer she immediately realized the implications for her future and was admitted after an overdose of paracetamol. She had no father and her mother's distress and reserved personality inhibited discussion between them so making the girl reluctant to go home. Refusal to be discharged, secret glue-sniffing and further threats of suicide were all ways of avoiding or masking the problem while also expressing anger at her fate and guilt about upsetting her mother. This was followed by a flurry of fashion consciousness, as though bargaining that if life were to be short it should be vivid. Family therapy slowly helped the mother-daughter relationship, but often it seemed like a race between restoration for them and the final onslaught of the disease. On the very last day of her life, the girl asked to go home. There could be no more pretending, but the two of them needed privacy. Later, her mother said 'That was the best night of our lives'. They were at last able to express what had previously been inexpressible, just in time.

THE SPIRITUAL NEEDS OF CHILDREN

It is only relatively recently that the spiritual needs of children have been recognized as needing inclusion when considering total child care [9]. The way that God is perceived may vary with conceptual understanding but a readiness to respond and relate to him personally does not depend on intelligence any more than does family affection. Even mentally handicapped children can show this, as can young children who come from unbelieving homes. That the advent of reasoning ability can for some quench simple faith, including that of many who care for children, should not negate the importance of this aspect of their lives for those whose spiritual awareness remains very much alive. It has been known for the trust in God expressed by dying children to rekindle faith in some of those who tend them. It is not uncommon for dying adolescents, whether or not they have had such thoughts before, to begin a search for spiritual certainties. We can fail them by overlooking this as a possible source of anxiety, though how help is offered will obviously vary with circumstances, culture and creed.

Professor Robin Becker tells how a young Arab boy was admitted to a Jerusalem hospital for cardiac surgery, but to everyone's surprise, during the preoperative assessment, he requested a Jewish skull cap and a kosher diet. Sessions with the child psychologist helped him to show, through his drawings, the terrible anxiety which had led him to set aside his own religious adherence. Like children the whole world over, his companions on the ward had fed him with horror stories, saying that he was fooling himself to think that his surgery would be corrective. Instead, his heart would be taken out and given to a Jewish boy. It took some time before he was finally, and with relief, restored to a Moslem lifestyle.

A 12-year-old boy with lung cancer had throughout his life been interested to talk about Christian things, although this seemed strange to his parents. When it became clear that he was getting worse despite therapy, he spent a lot of time lying with closed eyes and was thought by his mother to be asleep. She later felt that he had been sorting things out in his own mind, as after one such session he said to her, 'If I die, Mum, you're not to go worrying yourself and losing weight, I'll be all right, as I'll be with Jesus. It's you folk down here that will have to worry.' Eventually after discussion with him, the futile cancer therapy was eventually stopped, his quiet comment being, 'Well, my life is in God's hands: it's up to him what happens now.' Spiritual supporters were as important to him then as was any palliative medication, and his serenity so influenced his parents that they, too, came to share his Christian faith. This was no empty creed but an evidently real relationship, bringing another dimension of comfort into their lives as they lost their son.

CONCLUSION

Those who are concerned in the care of a dying child, whether unavoidably as family or from choice as professionals, need to familiarize themselves with the way that children of different age groups think about life and death issues [10]. It is possible to make matters worse for a child by expressing something important in a way not attuned to that child's conceptual understanding. Though we will not always get it right, an attitude of affectionate concern will encourage the patient and enlighten the carers. It helps to be able, imaginatively, to enter such a child's mind, always remembering that experience will have sharpened intelligence. Yet a child's priority at any age is for personal care and this will be of greatest comfort when dying. Whenever possible, this recognition should encourage us to enable each child of whatever age, whose death is anticipated, to experience from those near and dear, love and understanding right to the end.

REFERENCES

1. Shaffer, D.R. (1985) *Developmental Psychology: Theory, Research and Applications*, Wadsworth, Belmont, Ca.
2. Lynch, M. ii (1975) Health and child abuse. *Lancet*, **iii**, 317–19.
3. Field, T.M. (1985) Neonatal perception of people: maturational and individual differences, in *Social Perception in Infants* (eds T.M. Field and N.A. Fox), Ablex Publishing Corporation, New Jersey.
4. Delight, E., Goodall, J. and Jones, S.W. (1991) What do parents expect antenatally and do babies teach them? *Archives of Disease in Childhood*, **66**, 1309–14.
5. Delight, E. and Goodall, J. (1990) *Love and Loss: Conversations with Parents of Babies with Spina Bifida Managed without surgery, 1971–1981*, MacKeith Press, London.
6. Campbell, R. (1977) *How to Really Love your Child*, Scripture Press Publications, Wheaton, Ill.
7. Cotton, M., Cotton, G. and Goodall, J. (1981) A brother dies at home. *Maternal and Child Health*, **6**, 288–92.
8. Kubler-Ross, E. (1970) *On Death and Dying*, Tavistock Publications Ltd, London.
9. Shelley, J.A. (ed.) (1984) *Spiritual Need of Children*, Scripture Union, London.
10. Wells, R. (1988) *Helping Children Cope with Grief*, Sheldon Press, London.

CHAPTER 3

Talking about death – parents and children

Jack Cadranell

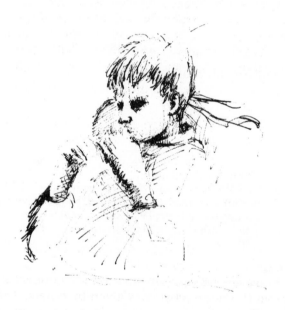

In the developed world the death of a child is an unnatural and greatly feared event. A diagnosis of life-threatening disease shatters the dreams and plans which parents had cherished for themselves and their child, It evokes intense emotions. Fear and grief, anger, guilt and despair may all play a part in this. Their world seems bleak and uncertain. It takes time for them to identify and mobilize their resources to cope with this situation. When their child is dying, all their worst fears become reality. For medical and nursing staff too the imminent death of a child may evoke feelings of anger, failure and helplessness.

Death in childhood has not always seemed so unnatural. Until the present century infant and child mortality was high. Medicine had little to offer to combat disease. The overriding question for parents was not *how* to raise their children but *would* they raise them [1]. Death was more accessible. People of all ages lived in extended families amongst settled communities and experienced the cycle of life and death at first hand: 'death was a public event and often took place in the presence of family, friends and children' [2]. In the eighteenth and nineteenth centuries childhood death was so common that evangelists sought to persuade parents that their first duty to their children was to break their wills, to save their souls, lest they should die unredeemed and, literally, be damned. Popular literature of the day invited children to consider the prospect of their own death: 'Are you willing to go to hell to be burned with the devil and his angels? . . . Hell is a terrible place . . . Did you never hear of a little child that died . . . and if other children die, why may not you be sick and die?' [3].

THE URGE TO PROTECT

Today, less familiar with death and free from the ever-present threat of infant mortality, we seek to protect our children and ourselves. Children are often shielded from events or discussions concerning death. They may not be able to visit even well-loved relatives and friends who are terminally ill. They are rarely allowed to attend funerals. Goodall (Chapter 2) has described how adults may lie to children to avoid discussing even the death of a pet: 'When a pet dies, it is not unusual for parents to rush out to replace it, pretending that the old one got lost or even trying to pass off the new budgie as still being the old one.' We worry that children have neither the emotional maturity to cope nor the breadth of experience to understand about death. We worry that we will not be able to contain our own emotions or find the right words to explain them.

Children, however, are very sensitive to the emotional atmosphere around them and to non-verbal cues given by others. They rely on the adults around them to interpret and help them to understand what they are feeling. What are they to learn if adults are prepared to go to great lengths to avoid the subject of death? What are they to understand when they sense distress but no one will explain to them what is happening? They are left with the questions, fears and fantasies which inevitably arise in their minds. Children are not always able to put their worries into words. Their distress may show mainly in the way they behave, and their behaviour may easily be misinterpreted.

Jane was a 6-year-old whose behaviour was causing problems for her family. She was being disobedient, throwing temper tantrums and doing anything which would draw attention to herself. She had always been a determined person but this was out of character even for her. Jane's father had haemophilia and had, in the past, been treated with blood products infected with HIV. He was dying in hospital of lymphoma, having suffered increasingly frequent spells of illness. Understandably, Jane's mother was struggling to cope with her own emotions and to offer her sick husband support. Jane was often looked after by her grandparents. No one had explained to her what was happening to her father. Daddy was ill but was 'getting better in hospital'. Jane could not understand why she saw so little of her parents and why, when she did see her father, he seemed so different. When she did express her upset in her behaviour it was seen as a nuisance. 'How could she behave so badly for us at a time like this?' The key to helping Jane and her family was to enable them to recognize and address her emotional needs and her need to understand her father's illness and prognosis. In the end Jane was able to join her mother in scattering her father's ashes, in crying and in remembering many of the events which had occurred during their short family life.

The lesson to be learned here is that, while we should not recklessly expose our children to personal pain and distress, we cannot protect them from it all. Life is inevitably painful at times and children need to develop ways of coping.

WHEN A CHILD IS ILL

The issues become more complex when the life at risk is a child's. If there is no easy way for a parent to learn that their child is seriously ill, how does one tell a child that they have a life-threatening illness? Many adults, parents and professionals would seek to protect children from this difficult news but for most children there is no real way to do so. One way or another they will learn the nature and seriousness of their condition. At some time they will be faced with a brutal reality. They will need to be well prepared.

Martin was 10 years old. He was returning to school for the first time after a long absence during his treatment for leukaemia. He was apprehensive but was looking forward to life getting back to normal. He was especially looking forward to seeing his friends again. He hoped they would be pleased to see him. He ran into the playground eagerly but became distraught when the first boy who recognized him said, 'My mum says I can't play with you. You've got cancer!'

HOW MUCH ARE CHILDREN AWARE?

Spinetta [4] discusses a number of commonly raised objections to talking to children about the possibility of their own death.

In relation to children it has been argued that they do not know about death, let alone the possibility of their own death. Even if they have suspicions about their own death they are better off not being told outright. In general it has been said that the adults around a child have the necessary strength to shoulder the burden of awareness and should not force the children to share it.

There is, however, much evidence that even children as young as 3 or 4 may have some concept of death and that by the age of 8 virtually all children are aware that everyone will eventually die [5].

Amongst healthy children the concept of death evolves gradually and there is a wide variety of attitudes and ideas. This process is speeded up when children are exposed to death at an early age. Sick children may have a sense that something very serious is happening to them which is far in advance of their ability to conceptualize or articulate it. This may include fear of abandonment and separation, of bodily harm and an awareness of their own impending death. Spinetta [6] reviewed literature which considered whether dying children were aware of their impending death and their experience of death anxiety. He concludes that children as young as 6 many express fears and anxieties which are 'real, painful and very much related to the seriousness of the illness'. He notes agreement in the literature that for fatally ill children under 5 'anxiety takes the form of separation anxiety, loneliness and fear of abandonment' and makes the important point that children may not always overtly express concern about impending death: 'Reliance on overt expressions of death anxiety that are easily observed can give a faulty or incomplete picture of the actual concerns of the fatally ill child and the psychological implications of the death threat for the child'.

Bluebond-Langner [7] and Lansdown [8] have each attempted to describe stages in the child's consideration of the seriousness of their own illness. Bluebond-Langner suggests five stages in this sequence:

1. Seriously ill.
2. Seriously ill and will get better.
3. Always ill and will get better.
4. Always ill and will never get better.
5. Dying.

Lansdown offers five more stages for consideration:

1. I am ill but I will get better.
2. I am very ill but I will get better.
3. I have an illness that can kill but I will get better.
4. My illness can kill my contemporaries.
5. I may die very soon.

He suggests that an important change takes place at stage 3 at which the child becomes aware of the potentially fatal consequences of their illness.

CHILDREN TALKING ABOUT DEATH

Children may express their feelings about death in a range of ways which will reflect their age and developmental stage, their experience of illness and death, their feelings for their families and their expectations of how their message will be heard.

Philip was 6 years old and terminally ill. He had always had a warm and demonstrative relationship with his parents. Now he had become withdrawn and uncommunicative, especially with his family. His parents worried that their relationship with him would be at its very worst during his last days. With paper and crayons he drew bleak, black and white pictures of death and loneliness – a boy lying in the road after being hit by a car, a wolf loping into the woods alone. He was able to talk a little about these pictures and to acknowledge that he was frightened of being left alone to die. This was enough to enable his parents to reassure him that they would never leave him and to re-establish the warm and open relationship they had shared before.

Eamon, also 6, was in the midst of treatment for a brain tumour. A family friend had recently died of a tumour. Eamon introduced himself to a new member of staff in the clinic: 'I've got a tumour but it's not the killing kind.'

Jenny, aged 8, was watching a pop concert on television and talking about a fellow patient who had died. 'Steven's lucky. He's watching this for free and soon I'll be there with him.'

Children can, at times, be breathtakingly frank. The American author Erma Bombeck was asked to write a book about children surviving cancer. She drafted out the first three chapters and took them, for critical appraisal, to a summer camp for children still under treatment. Around the campfire one evening she read out her chapters and invited the children's comments. At first they made positive noises, but then [9]:

'You just gotta make it funnier.'
'Right,' I said, jotting 'funnier' down on a yellow tablet.
'And the first chapter is all wrong,' they said.'
'What do you mean it's all wrong?'
They spoke with one voice. 'The first chapter should be ''Am I gonna die?'' because that's what everyone thinks about when they're first diagnosed.'

Offering children the opportunity to discuss and be informed about what is happening to them, including the possibility of their own death, is far from imposing an additional burden on them. It is giving them permission to talk about what is already on their minds. Without that permission they may be left isolated with their own fears, fantasies and misconceptions.

THE RIGHTS OF DYING CHILDREN

Gardner [10] has suggested four basic rights of dying children.

1. To know the truth about the probable outcome of their illness – or, since most children have already worked it out for themselves, to affirm the truth.
2. To share thoughts about dying – not just the probability of death but the many questions that follow. Does it hurt to die? If you're buried in the ground how do you get to heaven? Will you see Grandma in heaven?
3. To live as full and normal a life as possible.
4. To participate in the process of dying. To have a say in whether treatment continues or not, and in whether to die in hospital, at home or in a hospice.

Aronson [11], a survivor of childhood cancer, also calls the right to know the 'first and foremost right of a cancer patient', but adds an important rider.

> Now, it may sometimes be the case (more often, I suspect, with adults than children) that the patient does not want to know the truth or the rationale of his treatments. In that case, he or she has the inalienable right not to have the truth forced on him against his will. ... No one should be forced to confront a reality or an eventuality that he is not prepared to absorb.

PARENTS AND FAMILIES

What is required then is an open, continuous and respectful dialogue with each sick child. Ideally the child's family will promote and foster such communication, listening to his concerns, interpreting his feelings and setting them in context, supporting him as he comes to understand them and adapt to his situation. This is no easy task for a family under stress and struggling towards its own adaptation to living with life-threatening illness. Some families will never be able to offer their child this level of support.

Meeting the needs of the sick child is only one of a range of complex tasks facing the family. Serious illness interferes with all aspects of family life.

> The parents concur that the most difficult task they face is walking the narrow line between the amount of time spent focusing on the disease and its treatment, and the amount of time spent on one's spouse and the other children, on the continuation of life and living. [12]

The parents who adapt best are those who are able to share responsibilities with each other, who have broadly similar coping styles and who communicate openly with each other and with their child, especially about the illness [13]. Not all families, however, can tolerate such openness when facing the death of their child. Some may be able to confront the facts of the situation but not the emotional responses they provoke. Some are not able to communicate about it at all. This can pose real dilemmas for the professional working with the child and family, especially when the family will not permit others to be more responsive to the child's emotional needs.

Thomas, aged 13, was his parents' oldest child. His bone marrow transplant had been unsuccessful and there were no further realistic treatment options available which could cure him. He came out of the bone marrow unit without any of the optimistic atmosphere and plans which are the accompaniments of a successful transplant. He was morose and withdrawn but his parents were angry. They could not accept that he would not be cured. They began to contact treatment units around the country searching for one which would offer them more hope. They would not allow the hospital staff to discuss the situation with Thomas. Thomas took his cue from his parents. He asked no questions. There was a growing mismatch between his depressed mood and his expressed optimism about his future. The hospital team became increasingly concerned as they were prevented from offering him the physical and psychological palliative care they felt he needed. Thomas's parents moved him to two further hospitals within the few weeks before he died.

PROFESSIONAL SUPPORT

Every family will make its own adaptation to living with serious illness. This will reflect relationships within the family, its history and culture. What works for one family may not work for another. Each family will need at least the offer of professional support to achieve this adaptation. The task of the professional mirrors the task of the family *via-à-vis* the child. It is to listen to, understand and interpret what the family is feeling, to facilitate communication and to enable the family to identify and mobilize their own method of coping. This is not a time for the dogmatic imposition of views or of strategies. It is a time for support. The qualities most needed are those of genuineness, positive regard for the family and child and accurate empathy which have been identified in the effective counsellor and the 'inherently helpful person' [14] (see Goodall, Chapter 2). They are independent of the counsellor's theoretical standpoint. Truax [15] describes them like this:

(a) an effective therapist is non-phony, non-defensive, and authentic or genuine in his therapeutic encounter;

(b) an effective therapist is able to provide a non-threatening, safe, trusting, or secure atmosphere through his own acceptance, positive regard, love, valuing, or non-possessive warmth for the client; and

(c) an effective therapist is able to understand, be with, grasp the meaning of, or have a high degree of accurate empathic understanding of the client on a moment-to-moment basis.

To understand this is to realize that no one knows just the right thing to say to families or to children all the time. How one speaks to them and how one behaves with them is every bit as important as what one says. Listening carefully to them is most important of all.

UNDERSTANDING, LISTENING AND TALKING

Children do not exist in a vacuum. They are dependent on families which exert powerful influences on them and which, in turn, are influenced by them. Families have histories and are embedded in cultures which have helped to shape their values and their attitudes and feelings towards life and death and illness. These are the foundations upon which children build their conception of what is happening to them. An understanding of the family and its functioning is an essential first step towards talking to the child.

Listening to the child is the next step; learning first hand what they know about their condition, how much they understand of what has happened to them and how they feel about it. This is a time for patience. It is important to allow the child to dictate the pace, and to reflect and respond to the concerns and the feelings which they raise. Gathering, or giving, information is secondary to establishing oneself as an empathic listener, creating a safe and supportive climate in which the child can feel free to express feelings and may come later to raise more threatening fears.

Putting feelings into words can be difficult for everyone – especially so for young children. At times only their behaviour will give clues to how they are feeling or what they are thinking. Sometimes they may just look miserable or cry or have angry outbursts. When they do talk they may feel that what they say makes no sense. Accepting and giving words to these feelings lets them know that it is all right to feel angry or sad or bewildered, that no one knows the right words to say all the time.

There will be times when children do not want to talk any more. They may want just to sit quietly or to turn to some familiar and comforting person or toy or activity. They need to know that this too is all right, and that if and when they want to talk again someone will be there to listen.

Most adults worry about what to say if they are asked directly 'Am I going to die?'. There is a strong temptation to avoid the issue and to be falsely, and unhelpfully, reassuring. A response such as 'Is that something you've been worrying about?' can give the child permission to explore their thoughts and feelings about death and let them know that an adult is prepared to share this exploration with them.

For young children the overriding fear will be of loneliness and abandonment, of separation from their parents, from those they love and who love them. They need the realistic reassurance that they will not be alone, that there will always be someone with them. Many children worry that death will hurt. They may be feeling angry or frightened, ill or in pain. They need to know that dying itself is not painful and that their pain will have gone for ever.

For some children acceptance of their own impending death can bring a period of peace and reconciliation – of setting things in order.

Daniel was terminally ill. He was 13 years old. He had always been a difficult child, often in conflict with his adoptive parents. As he came to understand that he was not going to get better he talked at length with his parents. He decided who should have all his belongings after he died. He talked about his relationships with his parents and his sister and how he loved them. He died peacefully and his parents were able to feel that in the end things had been right between them.

THE PRICE OF CARING

Spinetta writes: 'How do you talk to children about their own possible early death from cancer? With great difficulty, with great concern, with care for the child, and with a heavy price on your own emotions and feelings' [4].

Caring for dying children is stressful for professional staff. The death of a child may arouse feelings of failure and guilt, or anger and overwhelming sadness at the loss of a much loved young patient. Confronting the emotions of parents and children can, at times, seem unbearable. Burnout is a very real possibility if carers do not take care of themselves. Acceptance of grief, anger and exhaustion and the opportunity to discuss these feelings with colleagues are the foundations of mutual self-care.

CONCLUSION

Despite advances in medical knowledge, cure is an unattainable goal in the care of some children. It is not the only measure of success. Good quality care is an attainable goal even when it has been accepted that a child will die. Helping children and their families to face that reality is perhaps the most difficult aspect of care. At its best it can enable even a short life to be lived with meaning and dignity right to the end.

42 *Talking about death*

REFERENCES

1. Newson, J. and Newson, E. (1974) Cultural aspects of childrearing in the English-speaking world, in *The Integration of a Child into a Social World* (ed. M.P.M. Richards), Cambridge University Press, London, pp. 53–82.
2. Judd, D. (1989) *Give Sorrow Words: Working with a Dying Child*, Free Association Books, London.
3. Janeway, J. (1753) *A Token for Children*.
4. Spinetta, J.J. (1980) Disease-related communication: how to tell, in *Psychological Aspects of Childhood Cancer* (ed. J. Kellerman), Charles C. Thomas, Springfield, Ill., pp. 257–69.
5. Anthony, S. (1971) *The Discovery of Death in Childhood and After*, Allen Lane (Penguin Press), London.
   Kane, B. (1979) Children's concepts of death. *Journal of Genetic Psychology*, **134**, 141–53.
6. Spinetta, J.J. (1974) The dying child's awareness of death: a review. *Psychological Bulletin*, **81**(4), 256–60.
7. Bluebond-Langner, M. (1978) *The Private Worlds of Dying Children*, Princeton University Press, Princeton, NJ.
8. Lansdown, R. (1987) The development of the concept of death and its relationship to communicating with dying children, in *Current Issues in Clinical Psychology*, vol. 3 (ed. E. Karas), Plenum, New York, pp. 37–47.
9. Bombeck, E. (1989) *I Want to Grow Hair, I Want to Grow Up, I Want to Go to Boise: Children Surviving Cancer*. Harper and Row, New York.
10. Gardner, G.G. (1977) The rights of dying children: some personal reflections. *Psychotherapy Bulletin*, **10**, 20–3.
11. Aronson, J. (1980) I may be bald but I still have rights, in *Psychological Aspects of Childhood Cancer* (ed. J. Kellerman), Charles C. Thomas, Springfield, Ill., pp. 184–91.
12. Spinetta, J.J. and Deasy-Spinetta, P. (1986) The patient's socialization in the community and school during therapy. *Cancer*, **58**, 512–15.
13. Burton, L. (1975) *The Family Life of Sick Children*, Routledge and Kegan Paul, London.
14. Truax, C.B. and Carkhuff, R.R. (1967) *Toward Effective Counselling and Psychotherapy: Training and Practice*, Aldine, Chicago, Ill.
15. Truax, C.B. (1971) The outcome effects of counsellor or therapist accurate empathy, non-possessive warmth and genuineness. *Vocational Guidance*, **7**, 61–79.

CHAPTER 4

Parents

Jane Thomas

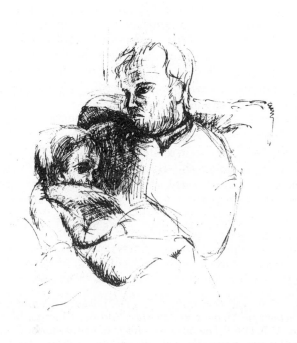

Our son Archie died in 1985, a few weeks before his sixteenth birthday. When he was 4 years old, it had been discovered that he was suffering from an inoperable brain tumour. During the 12 years after this diagnosis, there were periods of almost total remission interspersed with bouts of severe pain; there were hospital stays of varying length; there were different treatments and operations, and, when Archie was 10, there was a collapse followed by coma from which he was not expected to emerge. Emerge he did, however, to a further six years of vigorous and happy life. In describing something of that life and the effect of Archie's illness and his death and its aftermath on his family, I hope that those who care for and befriend terminally ill children and their families may find some help.

DIAGNOSIS AND PROGNOSIS

The first stage of a child's serious illness is usually heralded by the mother becoming aware that all is not well, and is followed by a visit to the GP. The difficulty for every doctor, in a case where no obviously alarming symptoms appear, must be to gauge the line between the anxiety of the mother and his own more optimistic assessment of the child's state of health. In making this judgement, two important factors should be borne in mind: first, to a mother, her role is to care for her child's well-being; therefore, when that child falls ill and exhibits symptoms which she finds inexplicable and which cannot be filed conveniently under the normal childhood illnesses of the measles or chickenpox category, she feels that in a certain sense she has failed in her role so she turns to the doctor as to an omniscient being and her only desire is for him to allay her fears. In this situation even an articulate, intelligent woman will subdue unconsciously the force of her own instinctive fears about her child, and allow them to be silenced by the wise doctor who is telling her that her anxiety is illfounded and that all is well with her child. Secondly, a mother, when she appears with her ailing child in the surgery, may seem to the overworked doctor to be fussy and tiresome, but nevertheless she should be listened to with greatest care. She is, after all, the person who knows her child better than anyone else, and her instinct where that child is concerned should always be valued.

In Archie's case, the maternal alarm bells started to ring when he was recovering from a fractured femur, following an accident while playing football with his dog. His recovery seemed slower than expected, and he started to refuse his food and to grow very thin. I accordingly took him to our then GP who was not only unsympathetic but lectured me severely. He told me that I was a neurotic mother whose fussy attitude was actually impeding my child's recovery.

Archie was an exceptionally intelligent and articulate child. It may be that on this occasion his friendly, bright and talkative manner disguised his real state of health and caused the doctor to dismiss my fears as ridiculous. This is a charitable view! Duly cowed and filled with self-blame, I took Archie home and, for the next few weeks tried, with increasing difficulty, to subdue my instinctive alarm bells which were ringing ever more insistently as Archie grew thinner. I dared not return to that scornful doctor: I never did, but instead asked a paediatrician friend who was coming to visit us if she would examine Archie. This examination led immediately to his admission to St Mary's Hospital, Paddington, for tests, and thence to the Great Ormond Street Hospital.

BREAKING THE NEWS

How can a consultant break appalling news to the parents of a sick child? Not easily, that is for sure. And yet it can be done in a way which is not entirely destructive for the parents. Many years ago it was customary for the parents to be told very little in detail about their child's illness and possible treatment: the lofty attitude was that it was not a good idea to regale them with medical details and possible alternative choices of treatment which would, most probably, be beyond their powers of comprehension. Now that attitude is a thing of the past, and most doctors recognise the importance of informing the parents as much as possible about their child's condition and likely prospects. Of course some people desire to know, or are capable of understanding, more than others, and it is for the consultant to judge how much detailed information is required in each case. But they should remember that, at this particular moment, the parents are bound to be in a state of shock and are therefore not best able to articulate all the questions or, maybe, to comprehend the answers, which will later come flooding into their minds. They are also, as described earlier, seeing the doctor as a powerful and omniscient being, and may be fearful of asking him to repeat things which have not been understood clearly.

It is a nearly impossible task for the consultant to get the balance exactly right, but there are three important points which he should bear in mind at this moment. First, it will give a huge and positive surge of strength to the parents to feel, at this early stage that the doctor is 'on their side' and that, however ignorant they, the parents, may be of complex medical procedures, they are nevertheless involved in the choices to be made with regard to their child's future treatment. It can also have a positive effect for the consultant at a later stage. The parents who have been made to feel from the beginning that the child's treatment is a team effort involving the parents, the doctors and the nurses will be in a far better position to monitor that child's condition and his response to treatment than the parents who have been made to feel that they have been pushed to the sidelines while the 'experts' get on with the job.

Secondly, the consultant who is breaking bad news will of course do so with gentleness and sympathy, but it helps the parents if, at this first, important meeting, that sympathy can be given a personal touch. This can be difficult if, as is not unusual, the consultant has probably seen the child only once or twice, and may be meeting the parents now for the first time. Nevertheless, a casual remark such as 'Your son/daughter obviously loves animals – we had a good chat about them this morning', or 'What beautiful hands Edward/Edwina has – is he/she musical?' will make the parents feel that the consultant has noticed that their child is a particular and special person and not just another number on a file.

Thirdly, there may be a feeling, when explaining a prognosis to a parent, that it is cruel to offer hope which will probably prove to have been ill-founded. There should always be a balance between raising false optimism and offering nothing but despair. Every parent in this situation will agree that the only totally unbearable emotion is knowing that something is desperately wrong with your child but not knowing exactly what. When the diagnosis is finally made and the truth is revealed, it is, however, appalling, preferable to the darkness of your own imaginings. So the parents should be given as clear and truthful an explanation of the situation as possible; but they should also, and in every case, be offered some shred of hope, even in a situation which the doctor privately considers to be hopeless. In Archie's case the initial prognosis was as bad as it possibly could have been. 'This child's future can only be described as grim' I read in his notes. We were told that he could probably only live for months rather than years (his brain tumour had been diagnosed as an optic glioma, affecting both the pituitary gland and the optic nerve of the left eye), that he would probably go blind, but that there was a very faint chance that radiotherapy might help in the short term. This hope was later to be triumphantly justified and surpassed. At the time, the fact that we were given that chink of light in an otherwise enveloping darkness gave a sense of purpose and an impetus which kept us going in those early days.

Every doctor knows that, even with today's advanced technology, it is not always possible to be exactly right either in diagnosis or prognosis. For every hundred or so cases which follow their expected course there is sure to be one which appears to confound medical expectations. It cannot hurt to give parents, at the beginning or during the course of what may be a long and difficult time, the hope that their child may be the exception to the rule.

Six years after that initial diagnosis, Archie became desperately ill. Scans showed that, after a long period of dormancy, the tumour had grown; he started convulsing every few minutes, and he lapsed at last into a deep coma. This time we were offered no hope. His consultants, who in the intervening years had become friends to us as well as trusted advisers, told us that it was very unlikely that Archie would ever emerge from the coma, and that, if he did, the inevitable brain damage caused by the lengthy convulsions meant that he would probably be severely mentally retarded and would certainly be blind. The previous damage to the optic nerves meant that he already had very little vision in his left eye and only tunnel vision in his right eye. After much heart-searching we asked for him not to be resuscitated when his breathing stopped. This decision was based on the premise that until now and in spite of his illness, Archie's life had been full of interest and happiness; now, if he was kept alive the future could apparently offer only a quality of life that would be unacceptable to him, and therefore to us.

Accordingly the oxygen was removed. But Archie did not stop breathing. A week later, sitting beside his inert form, I started to hum one of his favourite tunes – really as much to keep myself awake as to try to reach Archie through the coma. Suddenly, to my astonishment, a croaking but determined voice emerged from the bed, saying in an exasperated tone: 'Mum, not only are you out of tune – you're not even keeping time.' He then opened his eyes and announced that he liked the colour of the shirt I was wearing. So we had Archie back, and were to have him for nearly six years more, not blind and certainly no vegetable.

There is no censure implied in this story towards those fine doctors at Great Ormond Street; but it does suggest that even the blackest prognosis should be leavened with a little hope. When your child dies, nothing can make things worse; but while that child is alive, however tenuously, it can make parents feel a little stronger to be given a modicum of hope.

DURING THE ILLNESS

During the course of a terminal illness, whether it is a fairly short one or, as in so many cases, it is drawn out over many years, the professionals who have dealings with the family can offer support in so many different ways.

The right kind of advice

Some of these ways require a watching, listening presence rather than a well-meaning burst of advice. In this, the family of a sick or dying child has much in common with the victims of other disasters. Often nowadays, in any crisis, whether it be a gunman running amok in a peaceful market town, or a grievous air crash, we hear immediately that professional counsellors are hurrying to the scene; some hours later, these well-intentioned people are seen on our television screens, assuring us in caring tones that the victims of the crisis are coping well at the moment but warning that probably, in a few months' time, we shall see frightful emotional damage emerging. I do not believe that such warnings ever do much good. What does help is to have a friendly person at hand to sympathize, soothe and listen when and if the need arises. It is intrusive, patronizing and can actually be destructive if a professional encourages the victims of any disaster to believe that they are going to suffer in a particular way or at a particular time. The family which has been told that their child is terminally ill may be ranked with the victims of other disasters and should be recognized as such.

Unexpected stresses

So how can the professionals help? Perhaps at first by trying to understand some of the surging emotions which assail the parents, and by
recognizing that it is not always the time of acute crisis that are hardest
for them to bear. When a sick child is undergoing surgery, or is
suffering severe pain, or is hanging precariously on to life, there can
be terrible grief, rage and tension; but at such times there is action
too, even if it is only the action of sitting by a hospital bed, willing
one's strength to enter and heal that frail body. It is during the good
times when there is, maybe, a long period of sustained good health,
when the clouds seem to have rolled away for a time and there is happy
family life, laughter and holidays – all of which should engender calm
and contentment – that the child's illness can seem too much to bear.

Maybe it is that the human frame produces energy and adrenalin
to carry one through the battles of life, and then, when there is a lull
in the fighting, it becomes a petulant invalid demanding attention as
compensation for the effort that was needed to produce that surge
of strength; maybe it is simply that the division is too great between
the drama and tension of the life and death struggle on the one hand
and the mundane calm of everyday life on the other; and maybe too
it is the sight of the happy, healthy, laughing child, so great a contrast
to the pain-wracked figure of a few months earlier, which at these
times can bring to the surface all the bitterness and rage, combined
with a deep fatigue of spirit, which was dormant during the times
of high tension and drama.

For the doctors, the nurses and the professional helpers it is
important to recognize this, but not to warn parents to expect it. A
mother needs to be reassured that she is not going mad if, for example,
she feels like bursting into tears of misery at the sight of her happy
child running in an egg-and-spoon race, particularly when she
survived his recent severe illness or crucial operation courageously
and without breaking down. Hers may be a paradoxical reaction but
it is a normal one: this is the reassurance she needs and this is helpful.
It is not helpful if she is told beforehand that watching the egg-and-
spoon race is likely to make her feel miserable!

Marital tension

The strain caused to a marital relationship by the terminal illness of
a child can be, and often is, terribly destructive. It is another paradox
that their shared love for their child can actually drive the parents apart
from one another. Much has been and will be written on this aspect
of the subject, but there are a few points which can be of practical
use to those involved in such a situation.

First, not enough is generally appreciated about the sheer physical exhaustion of coping with a child's severe illness, particularly when there is no certainty how long that illness is likely to continue. Outsiders may be aware to some extent of the great pain and grief being shouldered by the parents. They are less likely to recognize that this grief and the strength needed to cope with it are also accompanied by, for example, the need to see that there is food in the fridge for the rest of the family, that other children may have to be met from school, their clothes washed and their dental appointments arranged, that the plumber has to be called to fix the leaking pipe, that contact with the office has to be maintained if the family's economic future is to be sustained and, perhaps most exhausting of all, that anxious friends and relatives have to be kept informed about the child's progress. Small wonder it is that the parent suffering from all these insistent demands will often turn in exasperation on the person nearest at hand who is, in this case, suffering from equal fatigue and is therefore the person least able to cope with this extra demand. This forms a seed bed for conflict and resentment.

Secondly, the two parents usually have very differing roles during the child's illness. Often it is the mother who is more involved with the actual care of the sick child while the father has to continue with his work. This can cause resentment from the mother who feels that she is shouldering the greater part of the burden, and from the father who feels he is excluded from sharing in his child's illness.

Thirdly, these differing roles can in themselves cause a widening split between the two parents. The mother, more conversant with every detail of her child's condition and treatment, may even taunt her husband with his ignorance, implying that it shows a lack of caring about his child; the father, after a bad day at work may seek to share some of his problems with his wife, partly to unburden himself and partly to shift the focus of her thoughts away from a total absorption with her child. This may be resented as insensitivity, or as selfishness, or as a lack of love for herself and the child, or more probably as all three. In this situation the parents themselves are probably not fully aware of all the underlying causes of tension. In each case their judgement is impaired by tiredness and strain, and this leads to more implacable resentment. This is where a friendly person outside the immediate family, and therefore not so affected by exhaustion and misunderstanding, can help to resolve such problems. And they can help best by listening endlessly, by not taking sides, and by offering only very unobtrusive advice.

Practical help

In a practical way, help can be offered on so many different levels. The friend who calls round with a family-sized casserole; the neighbour who takes over a weekly supermarket shopping expedition or a school run; the children's hospice which can give a real lifeline by enabling the parents to have space and time for their own needs, while knowing that their child is happy and in loving, experienced hands. It should not be forgotten that most parents of terminally ill children find it almost impossible to ask for practical help. This is not simply because there is a reluctance to admit their vulnerability and inability to cope; there is also a numbness, born of emotional and physical fatigue, which actually prevents them from seeing what might be done by others to help in this predicament. A sensitive person can help best by thinking themselves into the parents' situation and asking the question, 'What would help me most if I were them?' The answer is often an unexpected one: a drive into the countryside; a book or a bottle of wine; even a gossip about completely trivial things. In the middle of one of Archie's most serious relapses, an old friend called at Great Ormond Street, where I was spending day and night by Archie's bedside. She insisted that I leave the hospital for a quick snack at a nearby wine bar. As we sat down I asked wearily and automatically how she was. 'Frightful', she said. 'You would not believe what ghastly problems I'm having with the Gas Board … ' Her voice trailed off and, conscience-stricken, she looked at me in horror: 'Forgive me. How could I even mention such a thing while Archie is lying there … '. But suddenly, I realized that problems with the Gas Board were exactly what I most wanted to hear about and, relentlessly, I forced her to recount every horrendous and hilarious detail. Nothing else could have transported me so completely away from the hospital world I had been inhabiting for so long, and I returned to Archie feeling relaxed and refreshed. Only a perceptive friend could have understood that trivial gossip was what was needed at that moment.

SPOILING THE CHILD

It can be very hard for family and friends to behave towards the child as if life is normal. The temptation is always to offer treats and to satisfy every whim. It is important that everyone should be encouraged not to overindulge him with lavish presents, and, if treats are offered, to make them treats for the whole family. One so often reads in the papers of a group of kind and well-meaning people who have raised funds for, for example, a child in the late stages of leukaemia to be taken to visit Disneyland. Is that really what will give the sick child most delight? Is it not rather an occasion which will make a lot of people feel that they are doing something to help, but will not, actually, add much richness to the child's life? Does a child who is weak and probably in some pain really want to be taken through the turmoil of airports, and then exposed to the terrific hubbub and the crowds of a gigantic funfair? I suspect not. Perhaps those who are close to the families of very sick children should suggest that there are other, more subtle and more appropriate ways of enriching what may be a shortened lifespan.

When at the age of 10 Archie's health suddenly deteriorated, we were told that he could not survive for more than a few weeks, maybe a couple of months if we were lucky. He had always wanted to go to Scotland and he loved fishing. So we cancelled all our immediate plans, rented a cottage by a stream in the hills near Oban and, with his sister, Emily, spent a week fishing, messing about in boats, walking as much as Archie's health allowed, and watching the deer and the birds. It was a simple holiday, but for us and for Archie it was a golden time, and nothing could have given him greater delight. Important too was the fact that he was never aware that the holiday was in any way a special treat for him. Of course it was not easy for us to behave as if things were normal at the time, and shortly after our return from Scotland Archie became desperately ill, and fell into a coma, so that for a while it seemed that the doctors' predictions had been correct. However, as described earlier, he did recover, a shunt was then inserted into his head to help relieve the pressure of the tumour, and he was to enjoy several more years of happy and active life.

Looking back, we were glad that we had resisted any inclination to organize spectacular treats during what we had thought at the time were Archie's last few weeks with us. It is not only parents who find it hard to deny things to a child who is probably going to die soon. The rest of the family and friends should all, tactfully, be restrained from showering him with presents. It is, after all, every bit as important for a very ill child as for one in normal health that he should feel secure and like other children; it is also not unimportant that he should remain a lovable human being and not be transformed into a spoiled brat!

When Archie, who was musical, was 14, he set his heart on a 12-string guitar. He had played the guitar for years so this was no sudden craze. Much against our inclination, we suggested that he should save up for it himself, and so he did (helped, it has to be said, by cash presents at birthday and Christmas from grandparents who had to be forcibly restrained from buying it outright). At last the day came when the guitar was purchased and, after Archie died, I read in his diary for that day '**This is the happiest day of my life**'. I like to think that the great joy he had from that guitar was somehow enhanced by the fact that he had saved up for it himself. Archie was no saint, but he was a delightful human being totally lacking in self-importance. In spite of the inevitable attention he received because of his illness, he never became spoilt and this may have been one of the reasons why, all through his life, everyone found him so lovable.

Normality of behaviour

Moving on from this question of presents and treats, it is important
for the parents as well as for the child that doctors, nurses and other
professionals should always behave towards a sick child as though
he is absolutely normal both in health and in appearance. Gentle
humour and a calm, matter-of-fact tone can be more reassuring to both
child and parents than any amount of overzealous sympathy. If there
can also be some kind of spoken sign that the nurse or doctor
recognizes that this child is unique and special, the parents can gain
even more reassurance. A difficulty here, particularly on admission
to a new ward or to a different hospital, is not simply that the medical
staff concerned may never have met the child before; the sick child
may also be listless or fractious, his appearance swollen or otherwise
distorted by illness or drugs, he may be bald after radiotherapy or
he may even be unconscious. Such a child may not be a very appealing or attractive sight, and this can be frustrating for a parent. A mother
may long to say urgently: 'This is not really what my son is like; he
is bright-eyed and has thick, blond hair; he is agile and intelligent
and funny and artistic and kind and talented in lots of ways. Please
realize this and do not let his personality be hidden from you by the
way he looks now.' But of course she does not say this. This is the
same problem for parents mentioned earlier in this chapter, and the
solution is similar. Once again, it will be of inestimable help to the
parents at such a time if they can be given some sign that the doctor
or nurse recognizes the child's special quality. Perhaps they may
simply remark on the child's lovely smile, or ask about his particular
interests.

Several times during Archie's life, the opportunity for such recognition arose unexpectedly. On one such occasion in Great Ormond
Street, Archie, aged 10 and in a deep coma, had just been moved from
the main ward to a side room since he was not expected to live for
very much longer. My husband and I were sitting, silently grieving
beside his bed, when an unfamiliar nurse entered the room. 'I am
Ruth', she announced, 'and as I am going to be in charge of Archie
tonight, I have just come to introduce myself and to say how really
happy I am to meet you all.' We looked at our son's figure on the
bed, swollen almost beyond recognition by months of steroid treatment, breathing only with difficulty, and with tubes attached to hands
and feet. Happy? Ruth continued: 'Of course, it is sad to see him like
this, but so many people have told me what an extraordinary personality he is that I feel really proud to have been chosen to look after
him.' We could have embraced her. A few days later, during which
time this dear nurse always talked to Archie as if he were fully
conscious and alert, our son still in a deep coma, the consultant

neurosurgeon beckoned me out of the room for a chat in the corridor. I asked why, since I had been told that Archie could neither see, hear, nor respond to any outside stimuli, there was any point in leaving the room to discuss his case. 'I know that Archie,' said the surgeon darkly, 'and I would not trust him not to be listening to every word we are saying.' Another ray of sunlight and an assurance that Archie was appreciated as an individual, special person notwithstanding his present appearance.

Often other children, friends of the sick child, seem to have an ability to see past the distorted physical appearance to the reality of the person beneath. As a little schoolfriend of Archie's said furiously to her mother, who had unthinkingly remarked that Archie was looking rather fat: 'That is just the pills he has to take. Anyone with any sense can see the real Archie underneath, and he's not in the least bit fat.'

Coping with pain

The management of pain in a very sick child is primarily a matter for the doctors and nurses, and will be discussed elsewhere in this book. But it is very helpful for the parents if they can be consulted and their aid enlisted in the control of painful symptoms. So often with a child, even quite severe distress can be alleviated by alternatives to analgesics, and here the parents' understanding and cooperation is essential. Massage, relaxation exercises, autogenics and imaging can all be useful and can all be admirable ways for the parents and the child to work together to a positive and beneficial end.

Archie suffered bouts of extremely painful headaches, but disliked taking very strong analgesics because they made him feel as if he was losing control of things. We developed a technique of relaxation followed by visualization: the tumour was visualized as a lettuce (Archie's *bête-noire!*) being attacked and destroyed by the good forces of the body, here masquerading as pirana fish. This often seemed to work, and the pain lines round his eyes would disappear. Of course he did not abandon analgesic medication for pain, but he only took it when he decided that it was necessary, and never automatically at the onset of a severe headache. From the age of 7 or 8 the choice was always his.

Questions about death

This matter of control and choice involving the parents is also relevant to the difficult matter of a child's questions about his own illness and about death. A child who is or has been very ill will spend long periods in hospital, probably on a ward where other children die, and, in due course, the parents may well have to face the dreaded question:

'Am I going to die?' Possibly the best advice to parents who fear this question from their child is to temper honesty with a straightforward, rather matter-of-fact approach. After all, everyone dies sooner or later and nobody can possibly know exactly when they are going to die. People can be extremely ill and yet live to be very old. They can also be healthy and yet die after a very short life because they are careless about crossing the road. In Archie's case the question came after a long period in hospital when he eventually returned to school. After his first day back he announced with some relish: 'They prayed for me every day for three weeks. They thought I was going to die. Did I nearly die? Why didn't I die?' I heard myself reply: 'Well, you were very ill and I suppose some people might have thought you were going to die. But then you decided not to.' Archie seemed satisfied with that answer: he did like to feel that he was in control of things.

Siblings

This chapter mainly deals with the parents' view of the illness and death of a child, but it is impossible to do this without touching on the needs of other members of the family and, in particular, the siblings. When a child is dying, as when a new baby is born, the tendency of parents, anxious friends and relatives is to focus on that child, often to the consternation, bewilderment or anger of any brothers and sisters. The professional helpers can do much, both by reminding the parents to share this experience with their other children, and by example, to alleviate this tendency. Archie's sister, Emily, was 3 years older than him, and was therefore 13 when he was in a coma and, as has been described earlier, not expected to live for much longer. She was brought to Great Ormond Street so that she could see for herself that he was in no pain, and also, by implication, to say goodbye to him. She came into the room in great trepidation to be greeted cheerfully by Nurse Ruth: 'So this is Emily. I am pleased to have you here. I gather you are studying biology at school, so you are going to be a great help in looking after Archie. I am just about to change his drip, so if you could just hold this for me. Between you and me, your mother is a bit clumsy at doing this . . . ' Those few words and the nurse's attitude, did more for our daughter than hours of reassurance and explanation could have done. In a moment she realized that Archie was in loving, capable hands, that she herself was valued, and that she could actually do something to help Archie, even in this unfamiliar hospital ward.

AT THE TIME OF DEATH

So far we have been dealing with the events leading up to and during the serious or terminal illness of a child. At the time of the child's actual death, things move into a different focus, and the attitudes of the doctors and nurses can be of inestimable importance. Of course, if the parents want their child to die at home, and if this is feasible, they should be given all the help and practical resources necessary. When possible, this is often the least traumatic and therefore the best alternative. But in many cases the parents cannot choose the manner or the place of their child's death. During the later stages of their son's or daughter's terminal illness they may plan or imagine how they would like things to be, but the reality is often very different from the imagined state, and there is no rehearsal for the death of a child. So whether a child dies at home, in a hospice or in hospital, the only guidance for the doctors and nurses involved is that they should follow, as far as is possible, the instinctive needs of the parents.

This may not be easy. The parents may be dumb or inarticulate with grief and the nurse or doctor may have to divine by instinct whether it is best for the parents to cuddle the child, to hold his hand or simply to sit silently by the bedside. They must be given the opportunity to do whatever seems right to them at the time. It helps too if the child looks as peaceful as possible, maybe dressed in his own clothes, and with intrusive monitors and drips removed as soon as they are no longer of essential practical use. Such details are important because, for better or worse, this is a scene to which a parent returns in memory, waking and in dreams, to the end of his or her life. This is not a sentimental observation, nor do parents often mention it, but it does seem to be an inescapable fact, and for that reason especially, the moment of death should be made as peaceful and as dignified as possible. It is customary to ridicule the Victorians for morbid tastelessness in their habit of taking photographs of children who had died, often lying, hands clasped, in a bed of lace pillows and surrounded by flowers. We realize now that they were not so foolish, although today the child is likely to be dressed more informally and in everyday clothes.

In our own experience the hours before Archie's death were rendered nightmarish by the most appalling administrative chaos and bungling. He suffered a severe and unexpected stroke at home, but it was not until 6 hours later, after a series of increasingly frantic phone calls from local doctors, that he was finally, and grudgingly, admitted to the nearest neurosurgical hospital. The place, the doctors and the nurses were all unfamiliar to us and we were actively discouraged from remaining with Archie. He died 12 hours after admission, I was with him, and the moment of his actual death was peaceful. I was grateful for that, but I should have been still more grateful if the hours leading up to his death could have been similarly free from tension, noise and fear.

Immediately after the death of a child, whatever the religious beliefs of the family, the medical staff should try to ensure that the words

'Rest in peace' have an actual as well as symbolic meaning. The parents should be given as much time as they want to remain with their child's body, and should also be given the opportunity to wash and dress the child themselves, or help to do so if that is what they wish.

If the child has died in hospital, it may be that now the parents will feel a need to take the body home, or, if they are involved with one, to the children's hospice, for a time before the funeral takes place. This is a natural desire and can help the whole family to start to adjust their feelings by being quietly together in familiar surroundings. And what can the attendant nurse or doctor do or say at this moment? This can be a daunting moment for the young or inexperienced medical staff. As in so many situations of great stress, actions can often help more than words, and the best advice is to do what you would instinctively do if the bereaved parents were your own relations. Be natural and not contrived. For parents, the death of a child is the greatest of physical losses. For a mother, that child has come from within her body, has been nourished by her and, with its loss, she experiences the actual loss of a part of her own body. It follows therefore that at this moment of such tremendous physical loss, what she most needs is a physical response from those near at hand. An arm around her shoulders, a hand grasping hers will do more to assure her that, however imperfectly, you are sharing her grief, than would a wealth of words. You are offering her a shared humanity, and that is what matters most.

With regard to other members of the immediate family, our Western society tends to avoid direct confrontation with death, and there may therefore be feeling that it will be morbid or frightening for a child to see the dead body of a beloved brother or sister. In most cases nothing could be further from the truth, and it can indeed be very helpful for a child of any age to see their sibling after death. We all know that the most terrifying fears are the unspoken ones. To see the body of someone beloved, lying peacefully on a bed, is not frightening. It is reassuring to see that there is no pain or struggle and that the face is smooth and tranquil. It is even more reassuring to see that the spirit or personality which gave that figure life has vanished, so that the body is now only a peaceful but empty shell. Many children, our own daughter included, have had cause, afterwards, to feel glad that they were encouraged to see their brother or sister's body after death. It means too that there are less likely to be later fears or nightmares about their sibling being buried or cremated. They can better understand that the grave or the urn does not contain the essence of their dead sibling. At the time of their child's death, the parents may be too numb to decide what may be best for their other children, and time for such decisions is necessarily limited, so a sensitive nurse may often be the best person gently to encourage the right action in each particular case.

Post-mortem

It is, unfortunately, very soon after a child's death that a doctor may have to ask permission for a post-mortem to be conducted. However alert and controlled a parent may be feeling, and a surge of adrenalin is not uncommon after the initial abandonment to grief, he or she is not really capable of assessing fully the implications of this request. Of course most parents will acquiesce readily in the suggestions of the doctor and will be eager to feel that their child's tragic death can be used somehow by medical science to help other children suffering from a similar illness. They are not however, in a state to appreciate what their own feelings about the matter may be at a future date, particularly if it turns out that the post-mortem involved cranial or facial surgery and the inevitable disfigurement of the body. The shock of such a discovery can return to haunt parents for many years afterwards.

Delicate though such a conversation must be at such a time, the doctor should always strive to indicate that, should permission for a post-mortem be given, there will be no outward disfigurement to the body or, conversely, which areas of the body may have some alteration as a result of a post-mortem. If the parents recoil or seem to be distressed by the idea of a post-mortem, the doctor should not try to persuade them, except in extreme cases of medical necessity. The future emotional well-being of the parents should be set at a high value when weighed against possible benefits to future medical knowledge.

The funeral

So, a child has died and there are practical decisions which have to be made at once. Immediately after the death, once the registrar has been informed, plans have to be made for the funeral. In our Western society, death is nowadays regarded as something to be abhorred; the end of everything we regard as good and desirable. The tendency is often therefore to get it all over as quickly as possible, and the lack of a set pattern of cultural procedure can be bewildering for the parents. In societies where religious or cultural tenets are the backbone of daily life, the ceremonies following death are laid down and followed as a matter of course. Mourning and all its outward rituals of dress and behaviour are observed for a set period of time, and the family may remain at home for a statutory number of days while friends call to grieve with them. Certain foods may be eaten at specific times, a recognition that meals have an important symbolic significance in the family life on sad as well as festive occasions. The sorrowing relatives may gather round the bier to sing or wail as custom dictates for the prescribed time. A Chinese friend told me of her childhood

memory of standing by the bier of a young cousin and being made
to weep for long periods for several days. 'My older sister pinched
me every time I stopped crying,' she recalled. 'I disliked that, but I
was never upset by seeing the body, and I was not afraid of death.
It was all so much a natural part of life.' For the Orthodox Christian
too, the congregation at a funeral gathers round the open coffin holding
candles. They, too, are recognizing the tragedy of mortality while
celebrating the certain glory of eternal life, and for them this reconciliation is the beginning of healing. For these customs are rooted in a
sure understanding of the needs of the bereaved and may be envied
by those of us who live in a more secular and more doubting society.

But those parents without an allegiance to any particular religion
may need a friendly helper who will indicate the different options
available, encourage them to plan for the type of funeral that seems
best for them and, above all, to make them aware that the choice is
their own personal one.

There is sometimes a tendency, immediately after a child's death,
for the parents to feel that they want to withdraw and to be alone,
rather as an animal retires to a dark place to lick its wounds in solitude.
This is natural, but they should be dissuaded from shutting out their
friends for long. On the evening of the day Archie died, a friend who
lived some distance away appeared unannounced on our doorstep,
holding out a bottle of wine. 'I've just heard,' he said, 'and I wanted
to be with you.' Such spontaneous warmth can do much to break
through the initial numbness and desolation. Conversely, some
bereaved parents have found that people avoid meeting them after
the death of their child, as if their loss has somehow turned them into
social outcasts. This can be an added hurt to an already grievously
wounded spirit. The parents need an outpouring of affection from
their friends at this time. It is a sadness to see the announcement of
any death, particularly that of a child, followed by the words 'No
letters, please'.

Most parents find, in the months following their child's death, one
of their greatest sources of joy is reading the letters of sympathy from
friends. Such letters do not only make the mother and father feel less
alone; they can also recall episodes of laughter and fun shared with
the dead child, as well as giving an assurance that their child will not
be forgotten.

There may be some parents who genuinely feel that they cannot
face anything but the most private of funeral ceremonies, and such
feelings must be respected. But in the long term, and whatever actual
form it takes, the funeral of a child which somehow combines grief
with a celebration of that child's life can be an occasion, the memory
of which gives enduring comfort and pleasure as the years go by.
Archie was buried after a funeral at the little country church where,

eight months earlier, he had been confirmed. The qualities which made it special for many were, first, our determination that, however much anguish and however many tears were still to come, Archie's funeral should be a joyful affirmation of his own courage and hope and happiness. Archie's godfather gave an address which opened with the words: 'Today, gathered here as we are, we are not unlike a test match crowd who are standing to applaud the outgoing batsman – sorry that he is out and yet grateful for the pleasure that his performance has given us, and, in Archie's case, on a wicket that many would have deemed unplayable. His innings was a brief one but it was full of bold strokes and great courage.'

Secondly, we had not expected, on a frosty January morning, that many would come to his funeral. We did not think that was important. But hundreds of people came, from all over the country, because they had loved Archie or been moved by his story, and we found that it was important. Later, the memory of the love and goodwill flowing from that crowd of people would give us unimagined strength and comfort. The spirit of celebration continued during the gathering that followed the funeral. People remarked that usually on such occasions people conversed somewhat grimly about the weather, the food, the state of the country, anything, in fact, to avoid mention of the deceased. But on that occasion everyone seemed to be talking about Archie, laughing or crying as they recalled episodes of his life, recounting his jokes, and reminding one another of his idiosyncrasies. Archie seemed to be very much present.

There may not be, in our secular society, any right or wrong way to arrange the funeral of a child but, for the parents, the presence of loving friends, the opportunity to celebrate the life of their child as well as mourn his death, and the compassion and good fellowship of loving human beings must combine as a strengthening beginning to the next phase of their lives.

AFTERWARDS

Western society, while offering a proper sympathy towards bereaved parents, does not want to dwell on such a tragic event as the death of a child for very long. Once the funeral is over, it feels, normal life should be resumed as quickly as possible. But what is normal life for the parents of a child who has died? Of course, in a sense there is no such thing. The very fact of a child dying is in itself abnormal. We expect our parents to die before us, perhaps our brothers and sisters, maybe our partners, but nobody in this affluent part of the world, expects to attend a funeral of their own child. It is reversal of the natural sequence and is therefore an event for which we are physically and emotionally unprepared. The parents, then, are likely to have to rely on their own resources more than do other groups of bereaved people. How can they best be befriended? And what are their earliest problems likely to be?

For the mother, it has been emphasized, the loss is physical as much as emotional, and many bereaved mothers accordingly feel an actual physical pain after the death of a child. In my own experience the pain in my womb was so acute that I suspected some dire abdominal problem, until I realized that it occurred only when I was thinking of Archie. This is, I suppose, comparable to the experience of many amputees who feel pain or tickling sensations in a foot or a leg that no longer exists. As with so many of the problems which afflict bereaved parents, the greatest help is the simple assurance that such feelings are not in any way abnormal.

Loss of identity

Less straightforward is the loss of identity felt by the parents of a child who has died. Of course, all bereaved people feel a terrible emptiness in their lives, particularly in the early days. Daily life becomes a series of small shocks as, at different moments, the realization of loss comes crashing again into consciousness. It seems that part of the brain can take weeks or months to accept fully what has happened, so that for a long time after the death one may continue to go halfway up the stairs to call someone down for supper, look up from a book to share an amusing passage, lay that extra place at table, or glance at the clock wondering why someone is late home, before the horrified awareness sweeps over one again.

With the death of a child the feeling of emptiness for the parents is all the more poignant. A child is not simply another inhabitant of the household. He needs from babyhood to be nurtured and planned for, and the parents' role is to feed, clothe and protect him, preparing him throughout his childhood to take the huge step into adult life. When a child dies, all the expectations that were raised at his birth are cut short and the parents are left with nothing. Their plans for his childhood, adolescence, school, first job, friends, maybe marriage and their hope of grandchildren, all have disappeared, and there is nothing to take their place. For the parents of a child who has been ill for some time, this loss of identity can seem total. The mother who has spent months or years planning her child's diet, medication, outings, hospital visits and special care as well as meeting all the other hundred and one family demands has probably not only arranged her daily life but has also modified her family's lifestyle to suit that child's routine. She may, too, have sacrificed her own career prospects in order to meet the needs of her sick child. His life has shaped her life and that of her family and, when he dies, what is left?

The point to make to any parent who voices panic at this time is that, though nothing will fill that empty void, gradually daily life will readjust itself so that the emptiness will seem less appalling, and, more important still, that there is no loss of identity. A wise friend, paraphrasing the words of St John of Chrysostom, told me soon after Archie died, exactly when I needed this reassurance: 'You were and are the mother of a son. The fact that your son has died does not make you any less his mother now.' Our daughter, too, 18 when Archie died, found that this answered her own problem of loss of identity. 'I had started to think that I was an only child,' she told me, 'but I am not. I am still the sister of my brother who died.' This may seem to be a mere convolution of words. No matter. It can lead to an acceptance that what has happened has altered the focus of, but not extinguished the identity of the parent or sibling.

So the parental role still exists, but it is now apparently deprived of its reason for existence and must therefore be channelled into other practical directions. In the very early days after a child's death, the need for making arrangements for the funeral will take up much of the parents' time and occupy their thoughts. Once this is over, just as they need to talk about their dead child, so the parents also need to feel they are doing something for that child as a kind of continuation of their caring for his practical needs from the day of his birth. This is not so easy. A mother can no longer wash her child's hair, iron his football shirt, make his school sandwiches, or do any of the other domestic things she always used to do for him. What can she do to ease the pain of this unfulfilled need for contact with her child?

Practical re-organization

One of the first practical things that needs to be done is to sort out the belongings: the clothes, toys, treasured possessions and books of the dead child. This can be a harrowing task. The dressing gown on the back of the door, the book by the bedside, marker still in place, the anorak with pockets full of illicit chewing-gum wrappers, the half-written notes to friends, the hoarded programmes or photographs, the sight of all these can bring a shattering renewal and realization of loss. Often this task falls to the child's mother, and everyone approaches it in a different way. One may feel a great urgency to depersonalize the child's room as quickly as possible. To wash and put away the clothes, shut up the desk and pack away the toys so that the frightful wave of grief she feels every time she enters that room is somehow lessened. Another may feel reluctant to change anything. Every drawer, every shelf, every collection of treasures must be left untouched, as if the child were away for a short time and will return in due course. Neither of these attitudes is wrong and both are understandable. There is no right or wrong way of behaving after the death of your child. But if a parent persists for a long time in a very extreme attitude towards her child's possessions, it may be helpful for her to discuss her feelings with a loving and understanding friend. Take the first extreme example, the parents who, in their overwhelming grief, will banish every remembrance of the dead child from their home in a way that can seem heartless to an outsider. It is not heartless, but it is the saddest way in which bereavement can affect parents. Such parents are, by attempting to deny that child's place as part of the family, also denying themselves all the joyful shared memories of their child's life. At the other extreme is the parent who turns her child's possessions into relics and her child's room into a shrine. This is understandable. A primitive part of every mother who has lost her child will want to cling onto objects which, by sight, smell or association are redolent of that child. This should be recognized and respected. Nevertheless, with time, these physical bonds will become less necessary and can gradually be set aside as the parents begin to re-shape their lives. Perhaps the house will be full and the child's room needed for a guest; perhaps, as the room is cleaned, a few objects may be moved or put away; maybe some of the child's clothes will be given away, or some treasured possessions given to his friends. This should happen gradually and only when the time seems right.

In Archie's case it was several months before I felt a sudden urge to clear his desk. A lot of tears were shed as I read and sorted letters, diaries, scribbled notes, and examined hordes of objects, deciding what was to be kept, given away, or resolutely consigned to the dustbin. But in the end, I felt very close to Archie and as if I had somehow passed a difficult stage of a journey. The same process was repeated at intervals with his other possessions. There was seldom much logic or planning involved. It was two years before I suddenly decided to throw away his toothbrush, and six years before his room was completely redecorated and re-arranged. Now, seven years after his death, Archie seems as much a part of the household as if he had simply grown up naturally and moved away from home. We have a large box full of his letters and specially personal things; possessions such as his radio and typewriter are in constant use; his ties and cuff-links are worn regularly by my husband; his bedroom is a guest room with elegant curtains and beautiful watercolour paintings. But the bookcase still holds a huge selection of adventure stories and joke books, a guitar stands in a corner, and Paddington Bear still presides, standing staunchly and benignly on the chest of drawers.

Memories and memorials

After a child has died, the parents may suddenly find that they are unable to recall their child's face. They can see in their mind's eye separate details of hands, ears, the sweep of hair across the forehead, the turn of a cheek or the curve of the eyelid, but they cannot put the whole picture together. This seems to be a fairly common experience. It is temporary, but, while it lasts it is deeply upsetting, and it is important to be reassured that it is only a kind of short-term, amnesia which will pass. Parents need to feel that they will always have a true and enduring memory of their child's appearance. Photographs are, of course, an immense help, and a collection of photographs looked at together will often give a more vivid impression than a single portrait photograph. After Archie died, I made a big collage of photos taken throughout his life, and this was unexpectedly beneficial. For one thing it meant long hours sifting through old albums, selecting and rejecting, and, in doing so, recalling often forgotten moments of Archie's life. Then the process of arranging the chosen photographs, and including background scenes with particular memories and specially loved family pets, engendered a closeness to Archie and a feeling that I was, in part, doing this for him. There are many photographs of Archie in our house, but this collage, hanging in the kitchen, most vividly recalls his vibrant and laughing presence. Parents can also find tape recordings and, nowadays, videos, to be precious reminders when a child has died: previous generations of bereaved parents had no such possibilities of comfort.

Parents may find a different form of comfort in choosing a tombstone or memorial plaque. They should try not to rush into decisions about design or choice of inscription. Taking time to select something fitting and beautiful will help to fulfil the desire to do something for their child. In my own case this became something of an obsession, and many and various were the sources combed for exactly the right quotation to embody Archie's personality. I overheard my daughter say to a friend, as we were about to set out on a car journey, 'I am afraid that it may take rather a long time to get there. My mother has become a bit of a gravestone fanatic and we may have to stop at every church so that she can leap out and examine the headstones.' But when, months later, we had finally decided on a design, we all felt that the time had been well spent, and that we had accomplished something good for Archie.

Many families decide to arrange a memorial for their child which will in some way benefit other children. They may raise funds for a charity dealing specifically with the illness from which their child died, or for the hospital or hospice whose doctors and nurses helped their own child to live life as fully as possible. Sometimes, when a child has died in an accident, the parents have used their own tragic experience to highlight areas of danger and have, doubtless, helped to prevent the deaths of other children. However this is done, and whether on a local or a national scale, such fund-raising can be a memorial to a child who has died, and can also give a sense of purpose to the parents who are re-building their own shattered lives.

Sharing the grief

And how else can the parents be helped during this re-building process? Not by being told glibly 'Time heals everything'. The loss of a child is not a wound that ever heals. What is true is that, gradually, the pain comes less often, the tears become less frequent, and the deadened spirit starts to respond again to sunshine, music and laughter. These things happen fitfully and not in any steady forward progression. Interludes when life has started to seem bright and purposeful again can be superseded with appalling suddenness by periods of intense and overpowering gloom. Husband and wife may find that their moods of alternating lightheartedness and depression do not always coincide. Of course they are grieving together for their child, but each is carrying a heavy burden of individual grief, and they simply do not have extra strength to carry each other's suffering as well. It is better far, and often easier, if at this time a parent can unload their feelings of misery and hopelessness onto a friend who is not quite so intimately involved with the family. It can be especially helpful to talk to someone who has experienced the death of their own child. Parents who have suffered in a similar way are immediately, and without the need of words, on the same level of understanding as the bereaved parent, and can give, by their very presence, an assurance that life does go on. Recognition of the strength given by shared experience led, of course, to the founding of Compassionate Friends, that organization which has given and continues to give understanding and support to many thousands of bereaved parents.

Age is not relevant

A word should be said about the tendency to assume that the age of a child who dies is somehow relevant to the amount of suffering experienced by the parents. There is no such link. A child may die when he is 5 days, 5 months, 5 years, or even 50 years old. The parents of a child who is stillborn or who dies in babyhood may not be left with such a huge gap in their lives as are those parents whose child has lived long enough to become an integral part of their daily lives. But, conversely, their hopes for the future have been extinguished at the start; they have been cheated of any real knowledge of their child as an individual personality, and they have no rich store of memories from which to draw comfort. There is no equation of suffering: there is only the certain truth that the loss of a child is a total loss for the parents whether he dies as a tiny baby, as a teenager or as a grown man.

Acceptance

So, life will not be the same again. But, and this is a crucial question, would the bereaved parents **want** it to be the same? Of course on one level they would wish to be happy and carefree and without the sense of crushing desolation. But, if they had had a choice, would they have chosen never to have had that child? Surely the answer is always No. Whatever pain or suffering was involved, that child's life was a bonus for his parents. This can, I believe, be the beginning of some kind of acceptance. The parents could not choose whether their child lived or died, but they can in some measure choose how that child's life and death affect the rest of their own lives. They can, if they choose, spend the rest of their lives in bitter sorrow. In extreme cases some may actually derive a sort of strength from wallowing in their grief and self-pity for many years. In so doing they risk exhausting the forbearance and affection of their friends. Or they can choose to let that child continue to be a part of their lives, with a recognition that although the child's actual physical presence is no longer there, his influence and humanity remains an integral part of the family. Of course there will always be moments of anguish: the sound of a child laughing, the sight of a small, blonde figure running with a dog, can, unexpectedly and with appalling suddenness tear at the heart; but, and with equal unexpected suddenness, there can come a surge of delight on hearing a half-forgotten song or a joke, or at the sight of a rainbow or dazzling sunset such as used to be enjoyed with special pleasure by the child who has died.

This chapter has sometimes described the life of parents after the death of a child as a journey. If this be so, it is a journey without a conclusion and without a map. It can take many different routes, and there are no prizes for accomplishing its different stages within a particular timespan or in a particular sequence. Like most journeys, it has pitfalls and setbacks and times when the going seems very hard. But with friends at hand to offer encouragement at the darkest times, and with the parents' own determination to let their child's influence accompany them along the way, it can be a journey full of interest and vitality, enriched and not diminished by the life and death of their child. A final word to those helpers who befriend the parents on parts of this journey. You will be most valuable and most valued if you can listen endlessly, encourage unstintingly, support lovingly, and be gentle and sparing with advice.

CHAPTER 5

Brothers and sisters

Linda Zirinsky

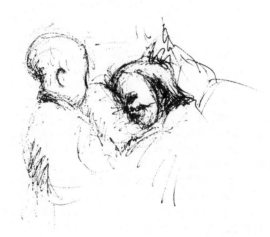

I only ever got angry with him once but I often felt resentment towards him for getting all the attention and then felt so guilty for feeling that way. I used to protect him and to care for him. I used to make sure that everyone else was coping but I could never ask for help with my own needs. I still can't.

This was how a capable, professionally successful woman in her twenties described her relationship with her chronically ill brother and its impact on her life. He had died several years before, but she was still struggling to deal with the remaining emotions. In particular she was trying to cope with close relationships, to let herself trust in and be cared for by others without feeling overwhelmed by thoughts such as 'I mustn't love him, he might die too. I'll be left behind. I must just fend for myself.'

I met this young woman as part of a research project studying the psychological adaptation of healthy siblings of children with a life-threatening illness – end stage renal failure. She clearly felt that having a brother who had been near to death many times and who had finally died, had had a profound effect on her. She was very gracious in not wanting to blame her brother. In fact she felt that often his bravery was the only thing that kept her family going. She was also clear that she had learnt much from the experience, but still she could see that in some ways she was emotionally disabled.

IS SIBLING DISTURBANCE COMMON?

How representative is this young woman of people in such situations? There are now several extensive and well-designed research studies which help us to answer this question. First, there are numerous studies looking at healthy siblings of children attending hospital clinics with a variety of chronic illnesses [1–9]. These studies show, in the main, an increase in psychological disturbance amongst siblings of chronically ill children, as compared to the normal population. There are many siblings, however, who are not disturbed, and positive adaptation is often shown.

The research has been rather heavily weighted towards cancer patients [1–4]. In all these studies healthy siblings of children with cancer have been shown to be at increased risk of developing psychopathology, as compared to the general population. In fact, the healthy siblings have at times been found to have a greater level of psychopathology than their ill siblings [2]. In addition, the level of psychopathology seems to be high whether the ill sibling is in a critical phase or in remission.

A child health study [10,11], surveying the general population, found that the healthy siblings of ill children had a twofold increased risk of developing emotional disorders as compared to siblings of healthy children. These disorders might consist of excessive anxiety, depression, fears, obsessional behaviour, etc. The healthy siblings of the ill children also had increased problems with peer relationships. However, certain problems were found not to be more common. These included conduct disorders (e.g. stealing, lying, aggressive behaviour), attention deficit disorders, social isolation and school problems.

Thus chronic illness is a risk factor for sibling psychological disturbance though fortunately the majority of siblings do not show any disturbance. The risk is increased when the illness is life-threatening. Similarly, studies of children who have experienced the death of a sibling show that they too have an increased risk of psychologial disturbance [12–15].

WHAT DO THE SIBLINGS TELL US?

What do the siblings themselves say about the experience of living with a chronically ill or dying child? One study [16] found that siblings of children with cancer spoke of losses such as disruption of interpersonal relationships, physical distortion of the ill sibling, disturbance in the routine of family life and alterations in the environment. However they also spoke of the gains they experienced, the opportunity for growth which the circumstances provided. This is an important reminder for professionals working with siblings. It must not be assumed that the experience is 'all bad'. The siblings often resent that, and seem to find it more helpful if they have an opportunity to tell the therapist how they have benefited from the situation too. Barbara Sourkes has worked psychotherapeutically with paediatric cancer patients and their siblings and describes themes which emerged in her work [17].

(a) Healthy siblings are often concerned about the cause of the illness. While they give one explanation which fits with the diagnosis they often also have another 'private' explanation based on guilt that they caused the illness or fear of the illness. It is important for the siblings to have a chance to express these fears.

(b) The visibility of the illness and the treatment required is often a concern to siblings, particularly at the time of diagnosis.

(c) Siblings may identify with the illness believing they too will be affected, alternatively siblings may feel guilty that they have been spared the illness or may feel shame, feeling that the patient marks the family as different.

(d) Relationships with parents may be marred by siblings feeling that the ill child is preferentially treated, that they are neglected or that the parents may be to blame for the child's condition. Encouraging parents to discuss these resentments with siblings may help considerably.

(e) Daily life outside the family with peers, and in school, may be a source of support for the siblings, or functioning in this area may be impaired because of illness preoccupations.

(f) Relationships with the ill sibling may be a source of difficulty. The healthy sibling may feel resentment, guilt and anger towards the ill sibling and the ill sibling may express considerable anger and resentment towards the healthy sibling. But an increase in protectiveness and caring is also often shown.

In a study which I carried out with 30 healthy siblings of children with end stage renal failure, the themes described above were also present [18]. I noticed that some children showed enormous openness about their difficulties, for example, one 10-year-old boy looked straight at me and said 'It's hard, you know, to have a brother who might die.' Another 8-year-old girl was able to say how difficult the time of diagnosis had been for her. Her brother had only been diagnosed when his renal failure reached end stage and therefore the shock was enormous for all the family. She spoke of how sad, angry, fearful and confused she had been and how these emotions gradually reduced over time. An 11-year-old boy described how he managed to deal with his anxieties. He said, 'It's like having two brains, you know, one keeps thinking of your brother and the other does things like school and football.' He was describing the defence mechanism of splitting, which we know is an important way for children to cope with painful issues. However, I also noticed that for many children a major concern which they had was to be 'normal'. These children did not speak of any difficulties instead they said they were 'just normal'. I attempted to explore whether these children had indeed managed to cope so effectively or whether they were in difficulties which they could not be open about.

Unfortunately, the latter appeared to be the case. They showed a considerable level of behavioural and emotional problems but were unable to discuss their worries. I even had the impression that their pain and distress was so great that they could not think about their worries and that this inability to think resulted in them exhibiting emotional and behavioural problems.

Two siblings spoke of having been disturbed but of recovering once they were able to think about and understand their situation. So, helping siblings to 'think about the unthinkable' (i.e. their predicament) is an important task for professionals and parents. This needs to be done gently and one needs to be very explicit that the siblings are normal, it is the situation that isn't.

ASSESSING THE RISKS

Are some siblings more at risk of becoming disturbed than others? It appears that low socio-economic level, poor marital adjustment of parents, parental depression, maternal anxiety, poor social support and low parent–sibling communication about the illness are risk factors for the development of behavioural problems in the healthy siblings [3,19]. Good family functioning may reduce the risk [20]. Being able to think about issues apart from the illness, being supportive of family members and being able to seek help where needed, are all characteristics of families with low levels of disturbance in the healthy sibling.

Siblings make great efforts to cope with their situation in a great variety of ways [21]. Unfortunately, we do not as yet know which of these ways are effective in reducing the risk of disturbance.

REDUCING THE RISKS

How can the risk of disturbance in a sibling be reduced when a child dies? Pettle Michael and Lansdown [12] studied 28 young people (aged 5–21) who had lost a brother or sister between 18 months and 30 months previously. The authors asked about the sibling's experiences around the time of the death, in particular investigating participation in events which have been postulated as aiding adjustment, such as: having knowledge of the diagnosis and likely fatal outcome; previously experiencing the death of a close relative or pet; having the opportunity to say 'goodbye'; having the sibling die at home; seeing the dead body; being given the deceased child's possessions; participating in the patient's care; attending the funeral. Siblings who participated in these events were less disturbed and had higher self-esteem than those who did not. Thus support was found for the notion that participation in these events reduces risk of disturbance following the death.

GIVING TIME

While we cannot take the pain away from children who have a terminally ill brother or sister, there is much that we can do to ensure that the experience does not have a long-term detrimental effect on their own development. One of the things which struck me during my study was how eager the healthy siblings were to meet me. I visited the children at home and they were often waiting outside for me. In one case the child had all his friends out on the street to meet me and show me the way to his house. The children seemed to appreciate greatly having some time with someone who was interested in them. This leads me to suggest that all professionals involved with a seriously ill child and his family should give time to the siblings. This time might include having the healthy siblings join in meetings with the family. For example, if you are going to ask how the patient is, why not ask the sibling too for their view on how their brother or sister is managing.

The siblings that I met in my project greatly appreciated being part of meetings with health care professionals. Two siblings who had two sisters with renal failure, each treated in a different hospital, were able to say that they much preferred the hospital that involved them in consultations with the paediatric nephrologist and in family discussion groups led by members of that hospital's psychosocial team. For primary care health professionals this task of 'including the siblings' is equally relevant.

Parents need to be encouraged to devote time to the healthy sibling too. Primary carers and specialists can be important in gently reminding parents about the needs of the other children. Professionals should help parents think about the needs of the healthy siblings, both in relation to their anxieties about their ill sibling and to their daily life. For example, spend time with parents talking to them about the often key issue of how much to tell the children about the illness. There is some evidence suggesting that open communication about the illness is related to less disturbance in the siblings [12,18], but this is not conclusive. In my research with siblings, there was a suggestion that the parent's attitude to informing was as important as the level of information the children received. That is, children whose parents had carefully considered what to tell them were less disturbed than those whose parents had not given the matter much thought, irrespective of whether they had decided to inform the children or not. Therefore helping parents think about the healthy siblings' needs may be very beneficial. Each of the other 'protective' factors listed by Pettle Michael and Lansdown should also be considered with the parents. They should be encouraged to carry them out and supported with them as much as possible.

While shortage of time due to the needs of the patient is often a factor preventing parents from thinking about the needs of their healthy siblings, it appeared to me from my study that another factor was important too. That is the parents need, like healthy sibilngs, to cling on to a view of themselves as a normal family and to invest the healthy child with the role of being normal. This means that if professionals ask about the healthy sibling they are often told that he is fine and they then feel that any further exploration would be unwelcome as it would unbalance this defence mechanism. It can be helpful to remind the family that while they are normal, the situation is not, and that a normal child's response to such a situation includes distress.

Primary carers will need to involve other agencies too in providing for the sibling. For example, they should not hesitate to contact the specialist services involved in the patient's care if they become aware of problems involving the healthy siblings. Such services usually have psychosocial teams attached to them whose scope often includes working with the patients' families.

In my experience, siblings are often deprived of a source of support which is much valued by parents and by the ill child – contact with people in a similar situation to themselves. Thus in the study which I carried out, all the parents and all the patients had contact with the other parents or patients but none of the siblings knew any other siblings of ill children. Some centres have set up groups for the healthy siblings of patients and these have been found to be beneficial [22]. While primary carers cannot run such groups themselves, they may be able to help put the siblings in touch with others, either through the treating hospital or through the relevant self-help group.

The well-being of the siblings is closely connected to the well-being of the other family members, so that all efforts made to attend to the psychosocial needs of the parents and of the ill child will have a positive effect on the siblings too.

REFERENCES

1. Cairns, N.U., Clark, G.M., Smith, S.D. *et al.* (1979) Adaptation of siblings to childhood malignancy. *Journal of Pediatrics*, **95**, 484–7.
2. Spinetta, J.J. (1981) The sibling of the child with cancer, in *Living with Childhood Cancer* (eds J.J. Spinetta and P. Deasy-Spinetta), C.V. Mosby, St Louis.
3. Cohen, D.S. (1985) Pediatric cancer: Predicting sibling adjustment. *Dissertation Abstracts International*, **46**(2–B), 637.
4. Maguire, G.P. (1983) The psychosocial sequelae of childhood leukaemia, in *Paediatric Oncology* (ed. W. Duncan), Springer-Verlag, Berlin.
5. Lavigne, J.V. and Ryan, M. (1979) Psychologic adjustments of siblings of children with chronic illness. *Pediatrics*, **63**, 616–27.
6. Tritt, S.G. and Esses, L.M. (1988) Psychosocial adaptations of siblings of children with chronic medical illnesses. *American Journal of Orthopsychiatry*, **58**, 211–20.
7. Vance, J.C., Fazan, L.E., Satterwhite, B. *et al.* (1980) Effects of nephrotic syndrome on the family: a controlled study. *Pediatrics*, **65**, 948–55.
8. Gayton, W.F., Friedman, S.B., Tavormina, J.F. *et al.* (1977) Children with cystic fibrosis: 1. Psychological test findings of patients, siblings and parents. *Pediatrics*, **59**, 888–94.
9. Ferrari, M. (1984) Chronic illness: psychosocial effects on siblings: 1. Chronically ill boys. *Journal of Psychology and Psychiatry*, **25**, 459–76.
10. Cadman, D., Boyle, M. and Offord, D.R. (1988) The Ontario Child Health Study: social adjustment and mental health of siblings of children with chronic health problems. *Development and Behavioural Pediatrics*, **9**, 117–21.
11. Cadman, D. *et al.* (1987) Chronic illness, disability, and mental and social well-being; findings of the Ontario Child Health Study. *Pediatrics*, **79**(5), 805–13.
12. Pettle Michael, S.A. and Lansdown, R.G. (1986) Adjustment to the death of a sibling. *Archives of Disease in Childhood*, **61**, 278–83.
13. Balk, D. (1983) Adolescents' grief reactions and self-concept perceptions following sibling death: a study of 33 teenagers. *Journal of Youth and Adolescence*, **12**, 137–61.
14. Stehbens, J.A. and Lascari, A.D. (1974) Psychological follow-up of families with childhood leukaemia. *Journal of Clinical Psychology*, **30**, 394–7.
15. Binger, C. (1973) Childhood leukaemia – emotional impact on siblings, in *The Child in His Family: the Impact of Disease and Death* (eds E.J. Anthony and C. Koupernik), John Wiley, New York.
16. Iles, J.P. (1979) Children with cancer: healthy siblings' perceptions during the illness experience. *Cancer Nursing*, **2**, 371–7.
17. Sourkes, B. (1987) Siblings of the child with a life-threatening illness. *Journal of Children in Contemporary Society*, **19**, 159–84.
18. Zirinsky, L. (1991) Coping with Adversity: Dealing with Illness in a

Sibling. Presented at 9th Congress of the European Society of Child and Adolescent Psychiatry.

19. Richmond, S.L. (1985) Factors influencing sibling reaction to childhood cancer. *Dissertation Abstracts International*, **46**(6B), 2051.
20. Spinetta, J.J., Murphy, J.L., Vik, P.J. *et al.* (1989) Long-term adjustment in families of children with cancer. *Journal of Psychosocial Oncology*, **6**, 179–91.
21. Walker, C.L. (1988) Stress and coping in siblings of childhood cancer patients. *Nursing Research*, **37**(4), 208–12.
22. Adams-Greenly, M. *et al.* (1987) A group programme for helping siblings of children with cancer. *Journal of Psychosocial Oncology*, **4**, 55–7.

CHAPTER 6

The extended family and other carers

Tessa Wilkinson

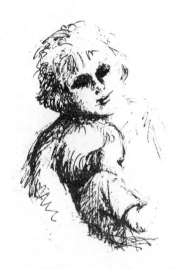

When a stone is thrown into a pool of water, it produces many ripples out from the centre. The ripples nearest to the stone will be deeply etched into the water's surface, and then in ever-decreasing depth they will move out from the stone. One small stone may disturb the surface of the water many feet away.

So it is when a child dies. Those nearest to the child will be most deeply affected and need most help to readjust their lives in order to live with the sad event. The ripples from the stone hitting the water are an image of the effect that a child's death will have upon the child's community. The death will affect many more people than the immediate family. The ripples will spread outwards into the community where the child lived.

It is of the utmost importance that those 'others' who may be affected by the death are allowed to voice their sorrows, and 'allowed' to grieve. Some will be affected more than others, but all should feel that it is right to be sad.

Of course, one must be aware of those who leap on to the 'grieving bandwagon'. Sadly death does sometimes seem to have a magnetic attraction to people, who seem to gain from 'having been there'. The risk here tends to be that the people who only turn up for the funeral, having not been around at all beforehand when help might well have been welcome, are those who disappear soon after the funeral, never to be seen again.

I shall focus on a number of the groups particularly affected: first, the extended family of grandparents, aunts and uncles, cousins and godparents; then secondly, those who have become an important part of the 'family' while the child was ill and dying – the doctors, nurses, health visitors, district nurse, home help and social workers; thirdly, those who have known the child in everyday life – teachers, school friends, family friends, dancing class, scout or guide troop, church community, local shopkeepers, parents' colleagues at work.

Of course not everyone in these groups will be affected, and certainly not in the same way. Some will naturally put the event behind them very quickly . Some, particularly those in the health care field, may have built up coping strategies over the years, not letting themselves dwell on the death for too long because they know another may follow soon after.

It is important to remember that it is quite normal that something as tragic as a child's death does affect our feelings. None of us is superhuman, and feelings of loss and sadness are not to be ignored. There are few people who do not experience them at some time in their lives. It is important for us to recognize and respond to them.

One of the first problems that we will have to cope with is our own feelings and thoughts about death, especially if we have experienced recently the death of a loved one. The death of someone else may bring back our earlier feelings of loss and grief.

When approaching a newly bereaved person we should put aside our own thoughts and feelings, and concentrate on theirs. That is not to say that we should not recognize our own experiences of pain and loss, but more that we should choose the right time and place to speak about it. 'I know how you feel because I have . . . ', is not what the newly bereaved want to hear. Even if the carer has experienced the death of someone they love, it must be accepted that different people will cope in their own way. We do not know how someone else feels; we only know how we felt in what we think is a similar situation. Each person feels pain and sadness in their own way.

Having accepted that when a child dies more than the immediate family will be affected, let us now look at the different groups in turn and see what particular reactions there may be, and how we can help each group to cope.

THE EXTENDED RELATED FAMILY

In this group I will include grandparents, aunts, uncles, cousins and godparents.

Grandparents will be grieving the loss of their grandchild, and may feel unable to support their own child, the parent of the child that is dead. The dead child's mother or father may turn to their own parents for help and not find it forthcoming. It is difficult for deeply grieving people to find the strength to reach out and help one another.

Because the child's parents may be used to getting support from their parents, resentment may build up. The parents of the dead child may feel let down. They may feel angry that their parents seem to be abandoning them just when they need them most. They may feel angry that their parents are grieving so deeply, when it is not their child who has died. Having someone who can stand back from the situation and help both groups of people to see what is going on, may be a way forward. When one member of a family is deeply grieving it is very hard for them to be aware of the other people around them and their feelings and needs.

One must never make assumptions about how upset someone should or should not be. Sometimes very close relationships can build up in the extended family. It may be that the grandparents cared for the child after school each day or during the school holidays. The shape of their lives, and their routine, will have been shattered by the child's death. They will need time to readjust to their life without their grandchild around.

Grandparents will often feel deep guilt at the seemingly outrageous situation, that their grandchild has died before them. The norm, and therefore the expected, is that grandparents die before their grandchildren; accepting that the reverse has happened may take some time. Often grandparents will say, 'If only it could have been me that had died. I have lived a full life, hers is only just beginning.'

Because people will frequently focus on the dead child's parents, the grandparents may feel that it is not their place to feel such pain and sorrow, and because they feel that unspoken message, they may try to bury their feelings. They will have to come to terms with the reactions of the people around them, who may assume that as it was not their child who died they should not feel so upset. But their grandchild's death has brought their own continuing future to an end; there may be other grandchildren, but that will not diminish the pain felt at the loss of the one who has died.

If the child has died of an hereditary illness, passed on from one generation to another, the grandparents may feel guilt that they were responsible. I have also known grandparents blame the other side of the family for their grandchild's death. They said, 'there is no problem in our family from that illness; it is our daughter-in-law's fault'. When this happens, deep hurt can be felt, and much help may be needed to heal the rift which may then occur.

It is not unusual for blame to be laid at someone's door. There seems to be a need to try to make sense of what has happened, and blaming someone or something may be how some people cope with their pain. It can be aimed at the doctors, the family or even God. Often it will be expressed in anger, with many 'if onlys'. 'If only the doctors had done this or the hospital that . . . '. This is often an intense and frightening time, and reassurance and love will be needed to help them survive.

An aunt or uncle might have spent many happy hours with the dead child; perhaps they have gone on holiday with the family. They could have been involved in supportive care while the child was ill. They may feel many of the same feelings as the grandparents.

A godparent may have very particular problems. As well as usually being a close family friend, a godparent has made promises about the child's future which he or she will now be unable to fulfil. Often faith may be particularly challenged when a child dies, and it may be that as well as having many unanswered questions of their own, because of their role in the child's life parents may ask them for answers to their own religious doubts.

Godparents and other family friends may have a child of the same age as the dead child, because the families all grew up together. These friends may have the difficult dilemma of not knowing how helpful it is to the grieving family to come around with their own children. Will seeing the dead child's friends give the family more pain, or will they be pleased to see the child, and want children around them? Will the godparents add to the bereaveds' distress by talking to the family about their own, well child: what she is doing at school, how much she has grown up? For someone feeling unsure about such things, the way forward is to ask the bereaved what they would like. If the two families have always talked about their children together, avoiding the subject could cause more pain than bringing the subject out into the open.

Friends need to remember that the bereaved are still the same people as they were before their child died. They have not grown horns or lost their ability to talk, so they should not be treated differently, but rather should be given the chance to talk about what has happened. If they cry, that is all right: the friends should not feel that they have caused the tears, it is just that at that moment the parents are feeling particularly sad. A newly bereaved person will be deeply sad most of the time. Giving them the chance to show their sadness will do them much more good than if the subject is ignored as if nothing had happened.

Another group that we need to be aware of is the child's cousins. Cousins can and do form very close relationships with each other. Because these family members are not always recognized as being involved, they may need permission to feel and acknowledge their pain and grief.

It could be that they find themselves feeling very lethargic and lacking concentration, a physical reaction often felt by the bereaved. Young people may be fearful of dying; especially they may fear that they could die of the same condition as the dead child. Being reassured that is unlikely to happen is important, as is being given the opportunity to voice these fears. It is so easy to change the subject when they start talking about it, and not to give them support and help when they ask for it. They could be very tearful and feel that their emotions are out of control. If this is happening, it might help them to find someone to talk to. YMCAs often offer counselling for young people. They will need someone who can help them to understand why they are feeling these emotions, and to reassure them that they will be all right; that how they are feeling is quite 'normal', and that grieving can be a helpful way forward.

Often there is uncertainty about how much to allow children to be involved. Should they go to the chapel of rest to see the dead child? Should they be allowed to go to the funeral? As is so often the case in these situations there is no one answer. If there is a strong request from the children to see the body, and if it is in good enough condition, I think the family should seriously consider what would be best for that child and his family. Often the idea of children being involved with this part of death is dismissed as wrong, without it really being thought about. Adults may well have their own fears about this time, which they will put on to the children. Allowing a child or young adult to see their cousin's dead body is not such an outrageous idea. The reality of the dead body may well be much gentler than the image that the child already has of death, often picked up from TV and videos. Seeing the body, touching it, and being allowed to see the 'deadness' may well worry the child less than wondering what it is like. Much love and support will be necessary; much time to answer questions and give information. It is the truth which will often give peace of mind.

I do not think that children should be protected from funerals; while the wishes of the family as a whole must be taken into account, if the cousins themselves want to be there, I think that they should be allowed to say their goodbyes. If they are to be present, then they should be told in advance what happens at a funeral; there should be discussion about the burial and about what will happen in church. If it is to be a cremation, they should be told what will happen to the coffin, and using real words, not euphemisms for death. Children are perceptive; they will know when adults are not being honest or are hiding something. Adults for their part should not be frightened to say 'I do not know the answer to that question'; but nevertheless it is important that adults try to find out the answers to questions and pass them on to the child.

THE EXTENDED MEDICAL FAMILY

The medical extended family includes consultants, GPs, nurses, health visitors, social workers, physiotherapists and people working in domiciliary care teams. Anyone working in a hospital or home care support team who comes into contact with dying children and their families may also be included in this category.

If a child has been ill for weeks, months or years, it is likely that there will be a wide group of people involved in the child's care, offering help and support to the whole family as well as to the sick child.

Today the 'professional carers' are often encouraged to keep their distance and not to become involved in their 'client's' or patient's situation. The reality is frequently very different. A special and very supportive relationship may be built up over a period of time. Because this does occur, and because 'carers' are human beings with emotions like anyone else, they will sometimes also feel the pain and sorrow of a child's death. Some may feel it more than others. I would want to stress that there is nothing wrong in having these feelings; it is not a weakness. They may be felt by the most senior doctor to the most junior nurse. These people are all normal human beings, and therefore have normal human feelings and emotions. Being 'professionals' does not make them immune to feelings of sadness or grief. It follows, therefore, that these feelings should not be suppressed, but recognized.

We all need to learn to understand ourselves, then we will cope much better with the stress of working with dying children and their families. We need to learn to recognize our own reactions, and allow ourselves to respond to them.

Troubles arise when we bury our heads in the sand and refuse to accept that we are not superhuman, but rather that we may all react in some way when sad events take place in our workplace.

Once we are prepared to say: 'I'm feeling sad' or 'I'm hurting' or again, 'I feel as if I have failed', then we can create a way of coping that meets our needs. Every person has to work out their own approach. Some will find a support group is helpful; others will find that one-to-one supervision is appropriate. If the workplace does not offer such support, then attention must be paid to creating it, by setting up a support group or making a contract with a friend or colleague to meet at regular intervals to support each other.

Some people find that it helps to do something physical, as a complete contrast to work, whether digging the garden, jogging or playing sports. Others find listening to music, or being alone helps them during sad times. Watching a sad film can be a helpful way to allow the tears to flow and to release tension. Whatever it is that works for you, use it.

Having a religious faith is a significant support to many people. Certainly, building up one's own philosophy and understanding of life and death is important. Without this we may be so wrapped up in our own fears and thoughts, that we can be of little help to others when we meet people who are having to cope with death in their own lives. There are books on the subject to be read, seminars or workshops to be attended. The life and death questions must be faced, both for oneself, and for those who are loved, especially if there has been a bereavement suffered recently in one's own life. One's own bereavements need healing before others can be helped.

Those who work with dying people need to allow death to be an accepted part of their lives. Those of us in the extended medical family need to recognize our own mortality, perhaps to write our will or even plan our own funeral. It is good to talk to those we love about our death and theirs. Do they want to be buried or cremated? Do we want to be buried or cremated? Is that a decision to be made by you or by the person who has to organize the funeral? Discussing this subject is not morbid, but sensible. Even if we do not know when, the one thing that we do know will happen to us is that we will die, and yet we do not readily talk about it in our everyday conversation.

When a child dies it may well be important that those who have been involved in the child's care should have the chance to say their 'goodbyes' both to the dead child by going to the funeral, and to the family. Going back to the family to say goodbye after the death is important both for the 'carer', and for the family. I have known many families who have been supported by a team of people coming to their home to help with the child's care, often for months. When the child dies they seem, often, simply to disappear. By omitting to say goodbye they are adding an extra sadness to that family. Families will say 'I thought that we had built up a special relationship over the months, and now they have just gone'. It is important that the 'carers' find time to go back to the family to let them know the situation. If there is no possibility of going back again, then that should be stated:

'I have come to say goodbye, I will not be able to come again.' Although that is hard to do, at least the family then know where they stand. If they are given the impression that the 'carer' will pop in to see them sometimes, and that does not happen, that will hurt much more than a final 'goodbye'.

THE EXTENDED COMMUNITY FAMILY

The final group to look at are those who are on the outer edge of the ripple caused by the child's death. This is a big group, often including large blocks of people together. For example, this group might include a whole school, a dancing class, parents' colleagues, scout or guide troops or the church community. Their link to the child may not be very close, but the death of a child is such an unusual event today that people can feel affected by it even at a distance.

Schools have to decide how they will cope when a child dies. The death of one of its pupils will sweep through the school like a bush fire, so it is important that the children are given some factual information as soon as possible, so as to stop rumours spreading. The child's actual class should probably be told quietly in a small group together. The rest of the school could be gathered together and told what has happened. It is important that the parents of the children have been forewarned and can therefore answer questions which may arise at home. Because death is such a difficult subject to give definite answers about, and because everyone has their own understanding about what happens after death, there may well be all sorts of ideas flying around school. This is a golden opportunity to study death and let it become a comfortable subject to look at. There are a number of books on how to introduce the subject of death to school children which may well be helpful (see Further Reading).

Because death is very much a part of life, it should be something that schools look at as a general subject, and the children will then be much better able to cope in their own family situations when someone dies.

A class pet which does not live too long is a good introduction to the topic (I recommend goldfish). When the animal dies the children can explore what has happened and openly discuss the subject. They can look at the 'deadness' of the animal; they can discuss what to do with it; a funeral can be carried out. Having been given a reason to introduce the subject, teachers can take it further and study the topic. The 'death' words can be introduced. Every child will experience loss at some time in their life, whether through death or other life events. To have already shared in the subject with others will make it much easier to cope with at an unexpected time.

The ages of the children involved will have to be taken into account. Children, of course, will have a different understanding of death depending on how old they are. Younger children may well not be able to understand the finality of death. 'Forever' means nothing to a child under the age of 4 or 5 years old. Children of this age will feel more abandonment than grief. Their implicit trust that someone who goes away will come back will have been broken, and much love and reassurance may be needed. Children between 6 and 10 years will begin to understand that death is forever. They will also often have very frightening images of death, and so the need to enable questions to be asked and answered honestly is of utmost importance for this age group.

The more adolescent child will have a more 'adult' understanding of death, and will often have picked up adult fears which may need to be discussed and clarified. Whether the dead child's school friends should go to the funeral must be discussed with the family and the parents of the children. If the family feel that they want a quiet funeral with no children present, then of course this must be respected. However, if the family feel that they would like the children there, it is important that the children be given the option of going. With plenty of information about what will happen at the service, children are certainly able to gain from being given the opportunity to say goodbye to their friend. We must guard ourselves from protecting children from funerals just because we feel frightened ourselves. The ritual of the funeral plays an important part in helping the reality of the death to be accepted. If there is no possibility for the children to attend the funeral, then the school might consider holding a memorial service which the whole school could attend. By doing this the school is helping the children to say goodbye, and showing the parents of the dead child that they recognize what has happened and that they cared.

Setting up a fund to raise money for a particular project which can be named after the dead child is also a way to help the children recognize that the death has occurred. Other groups which the child had been involved in, cubs, guides, or dancing class for example, might be invited to join in with the fund-raising. Many of the illnesses which can cause children's deaths today will already have a national charity to aid research and to help other sufferers, and this might be a good focus for fund-raising.

Children may build up a fear about dying themselves. If a child has died a violent death, other children will need much reassurance and help to overcome their fears of the same event happening to them. If the child has died from an illness the children may need reassurance that they will not catch the same disease and die of it themselves. It cannot be said often enough that it is most important to give the children the opportunity to ask questions, and receive honest answers.

When a child dies it will not only be the children in a school who are affected. The teachers may also feel loss and grief. Because they are having to be strong for the children in the school they may neglect to allow themselves to grieve openly. It may be important to have a staff meeting to discuss what has happened and the ways in which the school is going to cope. Within such a meeting, it is important that individual staff are allowed to reflect on how they are feeling themselves. Speaking about their feelings in a group may be difficult for some, and they should be encouraged to find some support away from the school and to take time to reflect on what has happened.

A further group who may be affected by the child's death in an indirect way are colleagues, those who work with the parents of the dead child. It is quite possible that they will have never met the child, but they will have come into daily contact with the parents. Grieving parents are often seen as 'different' and 'difficult'. People do not know whether to speak about the child, or to carry on as if nothing has happened. They worry that if they speak of the child then this may make the parent cry. They often ask the parents how they are in a way which does not give them the opportunity to answer honestly. If one is asked, 'Feeling better today?', it is difficult to answer 'No'. The way the question is put has an unspoken 'You are feeling better aren't you . . . I cannot cope if you are not'. If the colleagues can be brave and ask how things really are, and if they can ask whether the grieving parent wants to talk about the child, then everything can be brought out into the open and everyone will feel much more able to cope with a difficult situation.

Someone who is newly bereaved is not going to be functioning effectively. They will almost certainly be suffering from great lethargy. Grieving is very hard work and physically it can be exhausting. The grieving parent who is trying to carry on at work may be finding life very hard going. They may well need people around who recognize and accept this tiredness and lethargy and offer encouragement and help, not just in the first few days or weeks, but for months or years. It is important to remember that grieving does not go away quickly. People will often say that the time leading up to the first anniversary of the death is very hard, but that the second year after death is harder than the first. Most people will say that it takes months, leading into years, for life to come together again after a child has died. It is not unusual for people to speak of two or three years, and some people will need longer. People coming into daily contact with grieving parents must bear this in mind. The colleague who remembers that the anniversary of the death is coming will be much appreciated, because to have someone at work who remembers, is very special. Most people will forget, but just a note saying 'I remember and I am thinking of you', is all that is needed. It will cost very little in time but will mean so much to the recipient.

If the child's family are involved in a church community, they will usually find support and help there from the parish priest or minister and the congregation.

Coping with a child's funeral is always difficult for the person taking the service. Taking time to reflect on what death means and allowing oneself to face the big questions of life and death is of the utmost importance. Thankfully today, in the West, children do not die very often, but for that very reason it may be particularly hard for the person conducting the service. He or she may never have taken a child's funeral before. A child's funeral needs to reflect the sadness of a child's death, but also the laughter of a child, and getting the balance right can be hard. Taking the opportunities that arise to collect together some prayers or readings which might one day be suitable for a child's funeral service might well be worth doing. It will give the family some ideas for readings, poems or hymns which they might select for the funeral, making something which is very difficult a little easier.

Having helped the family plan the funeral, and having conducted the service and perhaps visited a few times, the priest or minister may need to reflect on how he or she is now going to help the family. Walking the road with a bereaved family is very difficult and time-consuming; keeping up with their mood swings, their moments of despair, their questions, their need to have their pain recognized and not brushed away, their 'if onlys ... ', is not an easy matter. If, on reflection, the truth is that there is not going to be the time really to support the family, it may be more appropriate to find someone in the congregation who could take on the continuing role. A bereavement visitor does not have to be a great 'expert'; rather someone who has some spare time to give to the family in an open and loving way, and someone who is good at listening and prepared to show love and care.

A church congregation must be sensitive to a bereaved family's needs. Sometimes a group of people who should be caring can be quite insensitive to the needs of the bereaved. They must try to see what the bereaved need, rather than dwell on how difficult they find the situation themselves. They should be the ones who stop and give time to speak to the bereaved about how they are coping, not those who cross the road to avoid them.

One of the problems that may be met by bereaved people who are Christian, is that other Christians may assume that a belief in a life after death removes the possibility or actuality of grieving. The truth is that even a great conviction that one's dead child is in a better place does not prevent a parent's much preferring to have their child with them here on earth. So even the message of hope in Christ's resurrection does not remove the pain for those left behind.

I return finally to my initial reflection on the ripples caused by the stone thrown into the pond. As we watch the ripples move onwards and outwards, we shall see that with time the surface of the water gradually calms and clears. So it is with bereavement and loss following the death of a child. Eventually, for most people, life calms down again.

How long that takes will vary from person to person, depending on how well they knew and loved the child. There is a gradual readjustment to the child's no longer being present. That readjustment does not diminish the loss of the child; the memories are still there and the experience of loving that child will always be present. Rather, it is the calming of the inner turmoil as those who loved the child learn to live on without them.

FURTHER READING

Duffy, Wendy (1991) *The Bereaved Child: A Guide for Teachers and Leaders*, The National Society (Church of England) for Promoting Religious Education, London.

Heegaard, Marge (1988) *When Someone Very Special Dies: Children Can Learn to Cope with Grief*, Woodland Press, 99 Woodland Circle, Minneapolis 55424.

Ward, Barbara (1989) *Good Grief. Exploring Feelings: Loss and Death with Under 11s*, Barbara Ward and Associates, 19 Bawtree Road, Uxbridge, Middx.

Wells, Rosemary (1988) *Helping Children Cope with Grief: Facing Death in the Family*, Sheldon Press/SPCK, London.

CHAPTER 7

Education and the sick child

Jean Lavelle

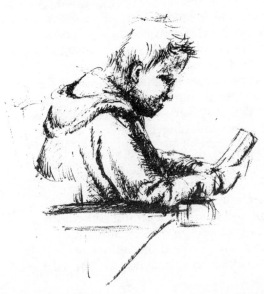

When a child is stricken with sudden and serious illness, education loses its place in the order of priority of need. For a while medical needs supersede all others, but sooner or later, it becomes apparent that formal education is an essential part of the child's growth and development as a person.

Continuing formal education is important for two main reasons. First, it is the right of all children to have the opportunity to develop their potential abilities to the full and enjoy the enrichment which education brings to life, however long or short that life may be. Secondly, going back to school re-establishes the normal pattern of life for a child and re-affirms membership of the peer group. Being with our contemporaries locks you into life. Family life and relationships are easier to handle when the daily routine is a comfortable and familiar one.

For a child who was born with a seriously disabling condition and for the child with a slowly degenerative condition, education is the door to a world of the intellect and spirit in which they can flourish despite their physical limitations. In recent years enormous advances have been made in the design of resources for children with exceptional needs. More importantly, I feel, attitudes have changed and it is accepted that education should be accessible to all, whatever their condition or life expectancy. This is now enshrined in the legislation of the 1988 Education Reform Act. The right to education is a normal human right which must be respected even when the situation of the child, because of sickness, is very abnormal.

How does one go about securing a continuing education for the sick child? The simple answer is to define the child's needs and match him to a service which can meet those needs. The answer in reality will probably be a compromise solution which will not live up to idealists' expectations but which will probably be the best match of resources to needs, available at that time.

Policies and resources for the provision of education to children with special or specific needs will vary from authority to authority. Details and titles may vary, but there should be a continuum of provision looking something like this:

1. Hospital services.
2. Peripatetic teachers and home tutors.
3. Special Schools for pupils with:
   (a) Moderate learning difficulties.
   (b) Severe and complex learning difficulties.
   (c) Behavioural and emotional difficulties.
   (d) Sensory and physical disabilities.
4. Ordinary mainstream schools with special facilities for specific needs.
5. Residential provision.
6. Mainstream schools with support staff.

The 1981 Education Act requires local authorities to name a Responsible Officer to whom parents can refer. This officer must make an assessment and a Statement of Special Need for their child. The name of this person is available from the office of the Local Education Authority.

During the course of a long illness the physical condition of a child may change and there may be long periods of remission interspersed with more critical periods when medical procedures or frequent therapy is needed. Continuing education in these circumstances may mean moving between two, or possibly three, of the options in the continuum of provision.

A key factor in the realistic understanding and best use of the available options is well-established and easy communication between the members of the interdisciplinary teams of medics, therapists, educationalists, welfare workers and parents.

Detailed knowledge of local provision and sensitive awareness of the child's needs at all levels is essential when deciding a placement. In balancing the child's medical, educational, emotional and social requirements, the voice of the parents sometimes get drowned. In order to be supportive, parents need to be confident that they know about all the available options, that their opinions are valued and that they have made an informed choice. When a placement decision is made, it is important for everybody concerned that there is commitment to the planned programme but also an awareness of other possibilities. It is comforting to know that there is another option available if the first choice placement proves to be unsuitable.

THE OPTIONS

Hospital services

Teachers in hospitals are usually funded by the Local Education Authority and exist in different forms. Their aim is to maintain the continuity of a child's education and avoid a total cut-off from the formal educational process. In the course of their work the staff also become consolers, supporters, advisers and liaison workers.

In a hospital, one would expect to find a well-equipped classroom, a class teacher, assistants and a small team of part-time teachers who visit the wards to teach those children who are unable to come to the school room.

The teaching task is complex. In a group of 20 children one might find nearly the whole range of chronological age and intellectual ability. The pupils here tend to self-select their own level of re-entry into coursework and are self-limiting in their on-task efforts. Liaison with the pupil's mainstream school is obviously very important. Cooperation between medical staff, parents and teachers from both sectors is needed in planning programmes, organizing resources and supervising the work. In this way, an individual scheme can be worked out which is geared to the child's capability but at the same time linked to normal mainstream work.

Home tutors

Home tutors are an endangered species and are not always part of an authority's team. Some authorities argue that the appointment of a home tutor delays a child's return to school. Others maintain that home tuition is an essential step in the gradual process of becoming emotionally and physically ready for the rigours of mainstream school.

Special Schools

Most Special Schools offer nursing and therapeutic services in an educational establishment which focuses very sharply on individual needs. The high ratio of staff to pupils means that children are taught in small groups, sometimes individually, and according to a programme which balances physical, developmental and intellectual needs. There is very close liaison with parents who appreciate the support, counselling and the feeling of security engendered by these communities.

Schools that specialize in the education of children with sensory and physical disabilities have a particular expertise in the early education, development and training of children whose potential abilities cannot immediately be assessed. Such children may be candidates for integration into mainstream school at a later date. These schools also play a very particular role in the recuperation and rehabilitation of children who have suffered neurological damage because of strokes, brain surgery or road traffic accidents. Short-term stays in such schools can allow a child a breathing space and a period of relative calm before having to cope with the tougher conditions of mainstream school.

Special Schools work hard at achieving normal academic standards and organizing liaison with the peer groups in mainstream school. Within restricted areas of the curriculum they can achieve above average results but they can rarely offer the full breadth of curriculum which one would hope to find in a mainstream high school. This type of school can, however, offer a specialized and self-selected educational programme to the sick child whose physical strength is seriously weakened and who needs constant nursing care and therapy. An enhanced quality of life can be achieved by defining and prioritizing aims and by using the educational process as a resource rather than an end in itself.

Mainstream schools with special facilities

Some mainstream schools have adapted buildings, offer the full curriculum and have some facilities for nursing and therapeutic care. In these caring but busy establishments the children need to be trained in a degree of self-management and to be confident enough to inform staff if their needs are not being met. Close liaison and cooperation between parents and school is essential. There should be a member of the teaching staff who has the special duty of maintaining this liaison.

Residential schools

A residential school is generally only available on public funding if there is no suitable provision in the local authority establishments.

Many of the residential schools are funded and managed by private charities.

The Special Needs Coordinator

The Special Needs Coordinator is the teacher in a mainstream school who has a particular responsibility for the care of any child with a defined special need. This teacher will liaise with the staff, the parents and all the other agencies concerned with the education and welfare of the child. The personal qualities and competence of this teacher are critical factors in the solving of problems and the smoothing of paths. Enthusiasm for the job and a talent for harnessing every available scrap of goodwill in their establishment are two of the most important qualities required. Goodwill, translated into action, overcomes a deal of negative bureaucracy.

Mainstream schools

If the aim is to return to the normality of life, then the neighbourhood mainstream school is the first choice from the options available. Returning to class in one's own school is obviously a more welcoming prospect than starting afresh in a new school. The environment is familiar and the staff well known. The people surrounding the child are old friends and classmates. It is easy to understand the daily routine. Although it appears to be the best option there can still be problems. What are the likely problems and what can we do to avoid them or, at least, minimize them? Let us start with the child's perspective.

RETURNING TO A MAINSTREAM SCHOOL

The child's perspective

Returning to the normal classroom after a prolonged period of absence is a daunting experience. Hopefully, some communication will have been maintained through cards, letters, tapes and visits from teachers and pupils. Exchanging bulletins and school diaries and keeping the absentee's files up to date with hand-out material are practical ways of keeping in touch and preparing for the return to the classroom. Appointing class 'watchdogs' to ensure that 'our mate' isn't missing out on anything is a useful ploy. The flow of cards and messages can be spasmodic and demoralizing for the recipient when it peters out. Regularizing the flow and, above all, maintaining it over a long period, will give confidence and security to the hospitalized pupil. Regular references to the pupil, anecdotes, quotes from the letters received and speculation about what input this particular person would have made to a class project will keep the class aware of the missing member and will keep their place 'reserved'.

When playing as a class, introducing a quiet moment which allows personal and individual reflection on the needs of the sick classmate may help to preserve existing bonds of friendship and prepare the ground for the absentee's return. This reflection can be turned to practical use by pooling everybody's ideas ensuring a warm welcome and a smooth re-entry into school life. An open discussion about these ideas may afford an opportunity to promote the view that continuous and regular support is perhaps more helpful than expansive, dramatic gestures of goodwill which are transitory and sometimes embarrassing for the recipient.

Classes tend to have their own chemistry and there are subtle changes when elements regroup. The classroom may not look quite the same and there will be evidence on the wall displays of experiences not shared. There may be new children and a rearrangement of places. School does not appear to be quite the secure place it once seemed: 'They've moved on without me – I don't belong anymore.'

A child who has had a prolonged stay in hospital develops some rather special relationships with adults. Informed medical discussions, serious counselling, deep spiritual exploration and friendly banter may have been part of the hospital experience. Suddenly, the adults appear remote and personal relationships with them are discouraged:

'He said, "Come and see me any time", but he's always looking at his watch and dashing off somewhere.'

Sparkling repartee in the hospital chat style does not seem to work either and the child is somewhat chastened when this is regarded as impertinence in school:

'I've hardly opened my mouth and I'm in trouble.'

There are new elements on the timetable, a brisk pace to the work and everybody in the old group has moved on to new work.

'I'll never catch up and they'll put me in group three.'

At playtime he is surrounded by an eager crowd of curious children firing questions at him about the nature of his illness and asking him about his future.

'What is going to happen to me? Is it true what Lee's aunty said? I don't want to tell my Mum and Dad – who can I talk to?'

Sometimes information about priorities does not reach some staff. This is more likely in high schools where there may be a hundred regular staff and some temporary supply teachers.

'The teachers get really narky when I remind them that I have to go out.'

'I told him I'd missed that bit but he said I would have to manage the best I could.'

'She said she would explain at the end of the lesson but there wasn't time.'

'I missed getting the homework down because I had to leave early. He thought I was skiving.'

'I wish I could tell somebody but they'd think I was whingeing.'

For the pupil who is already battling with the stress of illness and struggling to maintain credibility in the peer group, the casual dismissive or encouraging remark can carry a weight out of all proportion to its author's original intent.

'She said I'd have to buck my ideas up if I wanted to pass the exams. I'll never catch up ... they're three units ahead. I feel so tired ... what's the point?'

Equally, a teacher's attitude can signal to the pupil that education as a process is not confined to school.

'I got an A– for my theatre visit crit. She said that my ideas showed real insight and maturity and that my recent experiences had taught me a lot.'

Most teachers accept the dictum that education is a process of 'drawing out' but in practice their daily routine is a directed one which follows a programme of sequential work. Finding time to stop and listen, without showing impatience, will probably be difficult for the teacher but will be appreciated by the anxious pupil.

'I'm doing OK but when I get down I wish I could talk to somebody who didn't just push me on to somebody else. I want somebody to understand.'

The teacher's perspective

Introductory meetings between receiving teachers and the parents of a sick child are not always encouraging occasions. Often it is a first contact for a group of extremely nervous, defensive and possibly angry people. The parents, with the suffering of the child etched vividly on their consciousness, may perceive only vacillating and apparently callous professionals who are intent on outlining every possible difficulty and obstacle to their child's reintegration into normal school life. The teachers, with perhaps only a name and a hazy notion of the child's condition, may be afraid of very specialized medical care. Teachers are extremely wary of adding nursing duties to the ever-growing demands on them. They are also aware of their vulnerability to litigation if they involve themselves in activities outside their normal professional practices.

In recent years, with the advent of the National Curriculum and standardized testing, teachers have to work within narrower guidelines and are much more constrained in the allocation of time both for themselves and their classes. However, teachers are usually teachers because they care about children and many of them are also parents who will empathize with the plight of the sick child's parents and help them if they possibly can.

So, how can teachers use their teaching and management skills to help this child enjoy school life and learn as effectively as possible? A first step is to get to know the child. Even if the child is already known to the school, arrange a meeting for the child, the teacher and the parents. If at all possible this meeting should be at the child's home or on neutral ground where the parents are able to feel relaxed and not overawed by educational establishment procedures. Having met the person who is the subject of the case history notes and gained some insight into their present state of mind, one can study the professional data with greater understanding.

Getting hold of the facts

Communication between all the agencies involved in the child's care is essential. A realistic assessment of the child's needs can only be made when the medical, social and educational information is collated.

If the child is already a pupil of the school there should be no problem in acquiring educational information, but existing records may not reflect possible regression caused by illness or absence. Up-dated reports and assessment results may be available from the hospital, school or home tutor. This information should allow one to make a realistic projection of attainable targets.

Medical advice

Medical information is sometimes difficult to obtain and unintelligible to lay people when it is available. A clear account of the child's condition and the implications for the educational and physical management of that child should be available to staff who are expected to make an intelligent and sympathetic response to the child's needs.

It is also a salutary experience for a teacher to sit in on a medical team progress meeting where the management of the child's condition is discussed. Besides being informative this causes one to reflect on the priorities and perspectives of other professionals. Parents are also a good source of information and are usually happy to put teachers in contact with medical professionals who can translate the technical terms and explain their implications.

The hospital liaison officers and the district health visitors should be able to advise schools of any social problems likely to affect the child's education.

DRAWING UP A PRACTICAL ACTION PLAN

Meeting the physical needs

In order to avoid disruption when the child arrives, anticipate the probable needs by ticking off a check list. Does the child have any sensory problem?

Sight?
Hearing?
Speech?

Does the child have any perceptual or motor difficulties? Does the child have any physical difficulty which will necessitate extra provision in the form of:

Facilities in the building?
Special equipment?
Help from an adult?
Organized transport?

Does the child need nursing care or therapy in school?

Is there a contingency plan if the Special Needs Assistant is absent, if the transport does not arrive or if the child becomes ill in school?

Are there any school activities which would be inappropriate or harmful to the child?

Are there any infections which are particularly dangerous to the child?

Do the parents of classmates need informing about the need to report specific infections in their own children?

Does the child have a special diet?

Are certain foods forbidden?

Ticking a check list provides an outline of the child's needs. It avoids either over-dramatizing or minimizing the problem areas. One can now fill in the details and note any particular areas of difficulty.

It would be impossible to comment on every possible situation which might have to be addressed, but one important issue is the deployment of Special Needs Assistants.

Help from an adult

The adult helper may be a volunteer or a class assistant. Teachers need to supervise the adult helper very closely to ensure that the right level of intervention is being maintained. The function of the helper is to carry out those physical tasks which the pupil cannot do unaided. This usually means helping with toileting, carrying and setting up equipment and handling apparatus. The helper needs to be watchful and sensitive to the pupil's needs but not too obviously present so that they do not intrude into the peer group relationship. Maintaining the dignity of the person is an important element in this work. If it is necessary to cut up food for a pupil then let it be done discreetly and away from the table. Toileting arrangements should be as private and unnoticed as possible. There is a great temptation to do the work for the child. It requires tact and patience to be a good amanuensis and it is helpful for everybody if the teacher gives the helper a very clear definition of the task. Part of that task may be to work in groups alongside the assigned child so that help is at hand but not suffocatingly close.

Meeting the educational needs

Experienced teachers understand very well how to meet the educational needs of children. They also understand the restrictions placed on them by lack of time and resources. In the case of the sick child there are the further restrictions of interrupted schedules, the child's reduced vigour and the specific learning difficulties attached to certain conditions.

In the United Kingdom all children are required to follow the National Curriculum. Guidelines for exemptions have been studied but as yet there does not seem to be a definitive ruling about exceptions. One would expect that the National Curriculum would be 'disapplied', at least temporarily, in the case of a child with a life-threatening disease.

The aim in educating the sick child in a mainstream school is to encourage the child to follow, as successfully as possible, the normal educational programme, in the company of the peer group and in a caring and supportive environment. The immediate objective then is to organize and manage a programme of work which meets the curriculum criteria but which will not collapse if some parts or stages are not completed. If a child is re-starting a programme which depends on following a specific sequence of lessons, then the coordinator and the subject teacher need to pool their thoughts to produce a programme which will fillet out the essentials and enable the pupil to re-enter the normal programme without becoming too discouraged about the lost ground. Following curricular guidelines with maximum flexibility and recording results in such a way that the child has a sense of achievement will help to promote success. The child will only himself perceive a problem if the teacher does. If one has to admit to a problem then let it be in terms of coping with the organization of work and consult with the child about the best way to deal with it.

Cramming is not normally recommended but it can be useful if the child can cope with it and if it is restricted to a short period. A lot of follow-up work, while obviously valuable for reinforcing and internalizing knowlege, is not absolutely essential for the grasp of the concept. Written work can be very time-consuming for the child who has much ground to make up. Is there another option?

- Can one test by using Cloze procedure or just by a quick verbal check?
- If there is a folder of work to be produced, could the first drafts be in note form only?
- Are the teachers' notes available as photocopies?
- Is it absolutely necessary to hand-copy other pupils' work?
- Must the child work through an entire set of workcards before moving on?
- Would the staff be willing to get together to minimize written homework for a period to allow the child to concentrate on an intensive reading and viewing programme?
- How much of the teaching material is available as audio or video tapes? Could the pupil use it independently at home?
- Is there another group in school doing the missed 'hands-on' work?
- Are there staff available to give short periods of intensive tuition at times when the pupil is unfit for the timetabled lesson (e.g. rugby)?

Devising individual programmes is obviously a complicated exercise in organization and management. A whole school policy is necessary if the coordinator is to utilize all the talents of the staff in meeting a child's special needs. Working alone and unsupported the coordinator could not hope to cover all the child's needs.

Specific learning difficulties

Certain conditions entrain specific learning difficulties. Congenital birth defects, brain surgery or accidents produce brains which are functioning out of the normal pattern. Each case is different and it is dangerous to make assumptions about intellectual functioning until one knows a child very well.

Many people, and I include some teachers here, judge intellectual functioning by how well an individual can speak, read and write. Pupils with motor defects who cannot manage these tasks very well are assumed to have a low level of intellectual functioning and are grouped accordingly. They are frequently denied access to more stimulating and demanding programmes which they could enjoy. Recording by writing is an arduous task for the child with motor defects and this should be reduced to the absolute minimum.

Struggling for a word and then having to use such concentration in order to enunciate it or write it switches the brain away from the study of the subject. The thinking process needs to be a separate one, undisturbed by other demands. Some writing must be done of course. The pupil must still practise writing and course work has to be produced, but as many short cuts as possible should be allowed in order to take the tedium out of the task and preserve the enjoyment of learning.

Children with brain damage sometimes develop alternative short cuts in dealing with number problems which work, even though the method remains a mystery.

If a child has, or develops, severe perceptual problems then further help should be sought from the special education services or a Special School which caters for children with these specific difficulties.

Some conditions are degenerative and can involve both physical and intellectual functioning. Where the intellect remains unaffected, the breadth of education may become limited because of the physical weakness of the child. Some choices have to be made, and it is usually the child who will self-select some area into which he is willing to pour the last of his strength.

It seems to be very important to the self-esteem of these children to have such a goal. This goal is frequently a public examination, and however illogical this may appear to the teachers, the child should be supported in this as far as possible and without consideration of the final prognosis.

In these extreme cases the physical needs of the child become so demanding that they are usually beyond the scope of normal school facilities and the options of special or hospital school provision need to be considered. Such children can experience enormous relief when they relax into the atmosphere of the Special School. The normal peer group which has become an unwelcome benchmark for regression is now exchanged for a peer group in which everybody has some sort of problem.

In the case of a child with physical and neurological degenerative disease the educational problem is very complex. How does one appear to make progress while actually regressing? One can disguise the situation for a time by using differentiated material, introducing new apparatus and avoiding those situations where the child is most likely to fail. If the child becomes very distressed and anxious a Special School placement should be considered. Giving the child a chance to visit other establishments and offering an option will help to maintain a sense of self-management in a difficult situation.

Meeting the emotional needs

The whole purpose of getting the child back to school is to normalize their situation as far as possible. Therefore, the child should be treated like a normal school child. Rewards and punishments should be the same for all the class and the child should not be singled out for special attention.

Hailing the child as a hero or regarding him as a resident Tiny Tim* is not conducive to restoring the normal life pattern. Going to the other extreme and encouraging the child to overstretch himself is not helpful either. The aim must be to treat this child as normally as possible while being sensitive to those needs which are a direct consequence of the illness or condition. Parents cry 'I want them to treat him like a normal boy, but I wish they would remember how ill he has been'. The returning child may have a wheelchair, a stick, a catheter, a venous line, a hearing aid or may be bald. Some children may have a wig or headscarf to cover this condition. A child may be overweight or underweight because of drug treatment. School children are cruel in their mockery and marginalization of the child who displays any sign of being different. The teacher can help to defuse a possibly explosive situation by preparing classes and groups in advance of the affected child's arrival. The more children understand the illness and its effects the less likely they are to abuse the situation and hurt the sufferer. The class or group then identifies itself as a co-carer and becomes a support and a defence against the rest of the world. There is an unwritten contract to ensure that this child goes home happy. Embarrassing gaffes and careless unthinking remarks can be rendered harmless if the overall attitude in class is one of affectionate support. The members of these groups are also useful as prompters who remind teachers of the child's needs.

* The crippled child of Bob Cratchett in Charles Dickens's *A Christmas Carol*.

Specific information and details about medical conditions need to be treated with discretion. Consultation with parents on this point is important in order to establish how much the child knows and how much information may be passed on to the staff and other pupils. Parents sometimes take comfort in the fact that their child is unaware of the life-threatening nature of the illness. Frequently the child does know but keeps up a pretence in order to comfort the parents.

There are also several levels of awareness. One can understand an idea without being able to articulate it. Other forms of communication become more important at this stage. Body language and the comfort of a slight touch in passing can reassure a child without singling them out too much. 'I understand, I'm here and we're both getting on with life', one says without speaking.

If one's body is not behaving as it should, it is comforting to know that one still exists as a whole person in intellect and soul. The National Curriculum is prescriptive but it does still leave some element of choice of topic and one can take advantage of this to introduce studies which emphasize intellectual and spiritual qualities. Every teacher will have their own favourite sources of such material but, for sake of example, I would choose the work of Christopher Nolan, *Under the Eye of the Clock* and *A Brief History of Time* by Dr Stephen Hawking. The first is the autobiography of a boy with a poetic soul locked in an unbiddable body. The second is a science book which is incomprehensible to most people, including myself. One does not need to understand Dr Hawking's book in order to realize that the imagination and intellect of this severely disabled man have uncovered extraordinary clues to the mysteries of our universe. The vocabulary which had to be invented to describe concepts beyond our experience is a fascinating topic on its own. In pursuit of the awareness of ourselves as body and soul, the discussion of mystery is important because it introduces the idea of the transcendental without having to name God.

'There can't be a God; he would not do such things to innocent children.'

'What have we done? Why does God punish us like this?'

'My Dad says it's a load of rubbish. I've not to take any notice.'

While vehemently denying the existence of God, the child and the family may be looking for hope from a variety of alternative sources of healing and comfort. The child may find these puzzling and embarrassing. A general discussion about what people believe and how they express that belief might relieve the pressure on the child for explanations about the family practices. Sympathetic understanding of personal beliefs should be encouraged even if those beliefs cannot be shared.

Looking at how every culture throughout history has tried to understand transcendental experience will allow exploration of the ideas of mortality and immortality. God may invite himself to these discussions.

Healing is a difficult subject requiring sensitive handling. Raising expectations of miraculous cures is inadvisable but many people gain comfort and strength from spiritual counselling, healing services and pilgrimages and come to accept a wider concept of healing which helps them and their carers.

The myth of Psyche is another good starting point for discussion and drama. The drama lesson can be a good open forum and uncomfortable ideas can be expressed through the mouths of fictional characters. The role player does not feel embarrassed or exposed. A strong emotional and angry outburst is acceptable here. Wheelchair-bound children should be included in all forms of drama whether in the classroom or in performance. Wheelchairs can either be completely disregarded or made into fantastic props. They can be dragons, caterpillars, space ships, magic carpets, donkeys, aliens and mythical monsters. (Discourage the other children from using them as prams.) Always being narrator or prompter can be frustrating for the wheelchair-bound child.

It may take ingenuity and effort but there is usually a way to be found which will include the sick child in all the activities. This will do more for the child's happiness than giant teddies, trips to Disneyworld and footballs signed by the local team. If the school wants to raise money for an appropriate charity, then involve the child actively. It is demoralizing to be always on the receiving end of charity. Sponsored wheelies, sprout eating and spelling (not simultaneously) have raised sums in the past. If a role can be found for the sick child as a helper it is a great boost to confidence. Hearing lines, helping with reading and spelling are all useful activities, especially if it involves helping a less able child.

During the course of their illness, these children will have had experiences which have deepened their insight into the human condition. Their views, if they can articulate them, will add to the experience of the whole class. Let them be heard. However stoical and determined the sick child is to succeed in normal school, there are moments of physical and mental fatigue when the psyche is very vulnerable and a quiet moment with a sympathetic counsellor is needed.

Children seem to find this person themselves. It might not always be their teacher. It could be the caretaker, the secretary, the matron, a volunteer, a dinner lady or the group tutor. This person can become an important member of the care team and will pick up half-articulated anxieties which may not be expressed to friends, teachers or parents.

The peer group and one's position within it is very important to children, especially to adolescents, and the attitudes within the group can affect the happiness of its members to an extraordinary degree. The support and friendship of this peer group is so crucial that it should not be stretched beyond its tolerance by having too many caring duties imposed on it. A small commitment carried out faithfully is better than a ruptured friendship and embarrassed avoidance of contact.

THE SICK CHILD'S FAMILY

Brothers and sisters

It is sometimes claimed that the siblings of the sick child suffer more emotional trauma than the child itself. Whether or not this is true, they certainly need some special care. They frequently feel neglected and then guilty about being selfish. They feel a nuisance and hesitate to ask about their own anxieties. They have uncomfortable feelings of resentment towards the affected brother or sister which can cause them to act with covert cruelty. They wonder if the parents can possibly love them, the sick child is now such a paragon of virtue! They worry about the likelihood of contracting the condition. They need a counsellor and school is a good place to find one. Whether or not the sibling is attending the same school as the affected child, the relevant tutors should know about the family situation so that some arrangements for informal counselling can be set up. The normal routine of school may be a welcome release from a highly anxious atmosphere at home but concentration may be affected. Extra support and oversight of homework and public examination commitments may be needed since these areas will, quite understandably, have lost their immediate importance to the parents.

When a sibling dies the remaining brother or sister is sometimes afraid to express their own bewilderment and grief for fear of adding further distress to their parents. Grief can remain unexpressed along with the guilt of remaining alive while the 'better one' has departed. Opportunities need to be created which allow some expression of these inner anxieties through conversation, counselling sessions, writing or drama workshops. It may be some time before these channels are used effectively. The bereavement process is a long one and its effects may not manifest themselves until well after the period when it is expected that 'they will have got over it'. Sometimes it is only in adulthood that the grief of the bereaved sibling is finally expressed.

Grandparents

Grandparents are hurt for their own child and for their grandchildren. They are frequently desperate to do something to improve their grandchild's condition. If this energy can be directed into a practical support plan it can take a lot of pressure off the parents.

Grandparents can be patient supervisors of homework and sharers in the learning experience. School broadcasts offer a good alternative education if the child is confined to home and school coursework is sometimes available on video and if the school has a well-organized resources library it should be possible to borrow tapes for home use. Such material is much more valuable if watched with an adult who is prepared to comment and ask questions.

Grandparents also have a lifetime's experience on which to draw and they can offer their own curriculum of life skills, primary source history and scales of values.

Parents

Parents say that their emotions swing from iron determination to get the best possible education for their child to wanting to snatch up the child in their arms, dash home and close the door against the world. The teacher who is sensitively aware of the distress of the parents can help by listening and absorbing some of the stress. One cannot truly understand the parents' pain, but one can demonstrate a willingness to try. The professional advice can come later when the parents feel they can trust the teacher not to ignore their fears and misgivings. Interviewed parents relate experiences ranging from a school which became an extended family in its caring and sensitive support, to a school so grudging in its attitude that the parents could not have contemplated leaving their child in its care.

SAYING GOODBYE

If death happens, it needs to be recognized as a fact of life and acknowledged as a farewell. The teachers, emotionally affected themselves, may witness strange behaviour in the class and hear bizarre comments. Shock and grief cause ragged reactions which do not fit comfortably into preconceived notions of acceptable behaviour in these circumstances. There is a temptation to tidy the desk, remove all the child's work from view and return to normal routine as soon as possible. Normal routine may be a reassuring escape from uncomfortable feelings but at some point these feelings need to be expressed. For some children this may be a first experience of bereavement and their reactions may range through the whole sequence of numbness, disbelief, denial, anger, fear and guilt. Closing the classroom door and allowing the class to talk about their emotions and fears starts the process of healing. The questions may be difficult and the teacher's own inner resources may be tested.

It does no harm to shed tears or use body language to express sympathy and understanding.

Children may harbour feelings of guilt if they have been unkind or quarrelled with the deceased child and they may need help in the easing of this burden. Talking about the child, his work and talents and how he would have loved or hated the work in hand will allow memories to ebb and flow in a natural rhythm. Discussing the whole personality, faults and all, avoids canonization which can have a negative effect on siblings and friends.

Everybody needs an opportunity to say goodbye. An assembly in school or a service to which everybody is allowed to contribute their ideas is perhaps the most practical way to do this. Planning a memorial and raising funds for it allows grief to be channelled into positive action.

The family of the child will look for the support of school at this time. This duty is not an easy one and teachers are often afraid of saying and doing the wrong things. What can one do? The collated advice of experienced colleagues suggests that one should:

- Listen, talk, touch, be prepared to laugh and cry and sit quietly through the silences.
- Accept bizarre behaviour as normal for this person at this time.
- Don't say, 'It's for the best.'
- Invite parents to school, let them see and handle their child's work and promise to send it to them when displays are taken down.
- Maintain contact and be prepared, even after months, to discuss the personality and achievements of the child.

CONCLUSION

Teachers, through their normal training and experience, have all the qualities and skills necessary for the management and organization of the education of those children with special requirements. Their fears about being able to cope with the child's illness or incapacity are usually groundless but their worries about inadequate resources and support have foundation in experience. Material resources are important and one must battle for them increasingly, but the critical factor for successful integration of the child into the classroom is the warmth of the welcome and the attitude of the whole school. A school policy of goodwill and support is usually richly rewarded by shifts in attitudes, unexpected kindness from unlikely sources and an increased awareness of personal and social responsibility among the pupils and staff. This child is an asset.

FURTHER READING

Primary school level

Bergman, Thomas (1989)*One Day at a Time*, Gareth Stevens, London.
Bergman, Thomas (1989) *On Our Own Terms*, Gareth Stevens, London.
Varley, Sarah (1984) *Badger's Parting Gift*, Anderson Press/Armada, London.

Upper primary and high school level

Baron, Connie (1991) *The Physically Disabled*, Simon and Schuster, London.
Craven, Margaret (1967) *I Heard the Owl Call My Name*, Pan Books, London.
Paterson, Katherine (1980) *Bridge to Terabithia*, Puffin, Harmondsworth.
Shenkman, John (1990) *Living with Physical Handicap*, Franklin Watts, London.
Smail, Simon (1990) *Living with Cancer*, Franklin Watts, London.

Information and resources for teachers

Cancer Research Campaign Education and Child Studies Group (1990) *Welcome Back*, CRC, London.
Gatcliffe, Eleanor (1988) *Death in the Classroom*, Epworth Press, London.
Judd, Dorothy (1989) *Give Sorrow Words*, Association Books, London.
Kubler-Ross, Elizabeth (1983) *On Children and Death*, Macmillan, London.

CHAPTER 8

Spiritual care

Michael Kavanagh

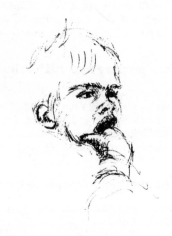

INTRODUCTION

The term 'spiritual care' can conjure up images of religious functionaries, of one kind or another, doing religious things. This may lead others within the caring professions to see such care as being a specialist field within which they themselves may have little competence. This chapter will, hopefully, show how all those involved in the care of a child in the context of his family can exercise spiritual care. The chapter will explore the issues from the point of view of how people make sense of their lives. This quest is one that concerns us all, and is therefore not simply the province of those who are 'professionally religious'.

It is vital that all people concerned with the care of the family should be sensitive to the ways in which the individuals, and the family as a unit, are making sense of their situation. Vital, because how people deal with the crisis of a child with a life-threatening condition will affect how they relate to the child, to each other and to themselves.

For example, if parents feel their child's illness is a punishment because of something they have done then this will have different implications for their feelings and behaviour than would be the case for a parent who viewed illness as 'just one of those things'. In the former case the carer would have to explore issues of guilt in some depth if the parent and the child are to be liberated to relate to each other in a new and more creative way.

This chapter will illustrate a way of approaching spiritual care from the perspective of enabling the child and family to 'make sense' of the situation. In talking of 'making' sense, it is clear that this task is active, engaging and ongoing. Sense is not given, but created. The format will be to look at the relationship the carer may have with the family, starting with the first meeting, through to the time of dying and into bereavement care. Towards the end of the chapter issues such as funeral arrangements and more specifically 'religious' care are discussed. Because of the limitations of space, this section is written from the perspective of being an Anglican priest and several years a chaplain at Martin House (see Chapter 11). This is clearly limiting, but the issues raised may be applicable to those who minister in a specifically religious way to those of other Christian denominations and other faiths.

For the purpose of this chapter, the term 'carer' will refer to the person who becomes involved with the ill child as a result of his illness. It will therefore most apply to those in the 'caring professions'. The children themselves are clearly part of a larger context which will be referred to as the 'family', and the children's key non-professional carers will be referred to as 'parents'. It is clear that this is only one, very traditional, pattern of life but the ideas explored may be translated to other contexts such as children in residential care or living with other relatives.

BEGINNINGS

The assumption that children do not die before their parents is one that is rarely spoken, but deeply held, in the relatively affluent parts of the world. The lower levels of infant mortality and the care that very poorly children receive away from their communities in hospital mean that most people, most of the time, are not forced to question this assumption. Many families with handicapped or terminally ill children describe their sense of isolation. This is caused not simply because of the lifestyle they are leading, which may include broken nights and regular spells in hospital. It is also cause by the fact that many neighbours, friends and family will tend to avoid them. Ostensibly this is because they feel that they 'do not know what to say'.

Another factor is that the encounter with a seriously ill child undermines their own sense of the world as being a safe, ordered place where, amongst other things, parents die before children [1].

Such an undermining of a sense of 'How the world is' can be even more profound for the parents and siblings of a child with a life-threatening illness. Each will have to make sense of what is happening and adapt their view of the world. This is often a long and difficult process that can manifest itself in a range of emotions and behaviours. It can seem quite daunting for a carer beginning to enter the world inhabited by a child and his family seeking to come to terms with death. There are no slick words or techniques that can make this meeting easy. Quite the opposite. It is possible to meet the family for the first time as the professional doctor, nurse, social worker, cleric or whatever and hide behind the things that these professionals do. This will establish a functional relationship which on a superficial level may be quite adequate. However, it will not permit the family to explore the deeper issues of meaning and the sense of isolation that they experience. To enter their world, much of our professional armour needs to be removed as we share with them, person to person.

Campbell describes such care as the 'medication of steadfastness and wholeness' [2]. Cassidy describes how such care involves the person simply as another human being, a fellow pilgrim, naked and vulnerable [3].

On first meeting the child and his family, it is important for the carer to attend to the whole context and not focus simply on the sick child. This can be daunting. It can often feel easier to go and 'do' something for the child, be it an injection or a baptism, and ignore the family as a whole. However, this can lead the child to feel isolated and powerless, the one who is always 'done to' rather than 'doing'. It also gives an implicit message to the family as a whole that the carer is there primarily for the child. At this early stage it is crucial that the carer is seen as someone who is, at least potentially, available for each family member. In this way the needs of the whole family are honoured and acknowledged. How such availability is communicated will clearly vary according to context, but attention should be paid to brothers and sisters in a way appropriate to their age, not simply to the adults. Talking to Teddy and looking at comics convey interest and availability to a child which is the foundation of spiritual care.

We cannot necessarily expect a family on a first meeting to suddenly talk in depth about the pain they may be experiencing. To cope with the disruption to their lives in physical terms and to the challenges to their belief systems, they will have developed ways of defending themselves from perhaps overwhelming feelings of sadness, guilt, anger or fear. It may well take time before they will trust a carer enough to let these barriers down. It may also need a different context. At this early stage it is an abuse of our power as carers to force members of a family to open up to us by very pointed questions; by doing so we remove more of their autonomy as people. It is tempting as professionals to try to do this because we want to feel we have 'got somewhere' or 'done something', yet we need to have the courage to wait.

At the end of the first meeting, as a way of conveying continued interest and concern, it can be helpful to make an acknowledged commitment to return. Depending on our role and the context, this may be 'in an hour' or 'some time next week'; the important thing is that the appointment is kept or the family is notified if you cannot get there. If you do not do this, they can either feel you are one more person who drifts into and out of their lives with no real care or commitment, or they can feel deeply let down. In either case, to regain trust at a later date becomes more difficult.

People with the obvious role of religious functionary can have the added difficulty, when ending the initial contact, of whether or not to do something 'religious'. Clearly each case will be different. Given the sense of powerlessness many families feel, it seems appropriate to ask them whether they want you to say a prayer, rather than just doing it because you expect it of yourself. Likewise, an act of blessing can seem rather formal at the end of an informal talk but, given particular religious affiliations on the part of the family, may be quite appropriate. However, if a prayer or a blessing is used, care must be taken with the words used. The family will undoubtedly listen very carefully and loaded words like 'healing' can carry connotations for them that are quite different from those you may intend. If such words are used, they need to be talked through, so it would be more appropriate to delay their use until the family know you better and you know them.

GOING ON

Facing the death of someone we love or coming to terms with our own mortality raises the question 'What is the point of life?' What is the meaning of life? It would perhaps be comforting if we could answer this question in purely rational terms. The ultimate expression of such a rational answer is the one found in *The Hitch-hikers Guide to the Galaxy* [4], where we are assured the answer is 'Forty-two'! But for most of us, meaning is experienced as a complex of feelings, beliefs and past experiences within which we have a sense of life having some sort of point or purpose. If we are asked to express our sense of meaning we may do so in the language of religious faith. So, for St Ignatius, life's meaning is found in the following words:

God freely created us so that we might know, love and serve him in this life and be happy with him forever [5].

But for many people, clothing life's meaning in words at all is difficult, and they would describe meaningful experiences – times when they felt life had meaning such as falling in love, the birth of a child, seeing a sunset, or listening to music. T.S. Eliot speaks of times when words simply are not able in any straightforward way to convey what we are trying to say:

Words strain,
Crack and sometimes break under the burden.
Under the tension, slip, slide, perish,
Decay with imprecision, will not stay in place,
Will not stay still. [6]

Even at times in our lives when we may feel fairly calm, trying to convey what we most deeply feel about that which gives life meaning can be very hard and encompasses not simply the rational parts of ourselves, but also the emotional and pragmatic parts. Our sense of meaning, the framework within which we live our lives, develops over time as a result of a complex interaction between our own psychological development and the experiences we encounter in the world. It is an attempt to give order and predictability to our lives.* However, it is very subtle; almost like the backdrop to the way we live our lives in that it is always there, hardly noticed, difficult to grasp, intensely personal and therefore hard to articulate. Given severe and sudden changes in the contours of our lives, this backdrop suddenly comes into focus because it seems as if what we have until now taken for granted is suddenly so no longer. The possibility of a child dying is one such experience. As carers we need to help people begin to review their sense of meaning in the light of this new and deeply unwelcome fact. In doing so, we too will be changed.

How can we go about this task? The whole area of listening is clearly crucial. This tends to imply a focus on spoken words, yet the listening required is more akin to openness, to the range of feelings being expressed by the person at both a verbal and a non-verbal level as well as to what is being evoked in us. Its meaning is not a matter of rational propositions. In being open to another who is struggling to overcome isolation and articulate meaning we need to be flexible. With adults, one way forward is through the use of metaphor. Metaphors may come up naturally in conversation as word pictures about how people are feeling, or they may be elicited by questions such as 'What does it feel like?' It is crucial that such pictures are remembered

* This approach may be found exemplified in the work of Miller-Mair [7] and Rowe [8].

by the professional carer because they provide a bridge between the internal world of the person who is hurting and that of the carer in such a way that real 'hearing' can take place.

A person may describe a picture, such as being in a boat in a rough sea, all alone, with no sign of land. A moment's imagination highlights the fact that their world has become unpredictable and isolating. Enquiring about how the person in the boat feels can show more deeply what is being felt – perhaps a sense of fear. 'Is the boat strong?': the answer to this may reveal the extent of a person's vulnerability. If the person were to say, 'I feel I cannot go on, I just want it to end', the depth of this cry and the action needed may be quite different in the case of someone who feels secure in their boat, as opposed to one who feels their boat is sinking.

Another person may describe being unable to feel; that their heart is stone. Exploring this in a gentle way may reveal that trapped in their heart are so many feelings that they would explode if they were allowed out. This shows a clear caution about how challenging conversations should be, and the need to spend time to allow the stone to develop small cracks to let the pressure out slowly.

Metaphorical language may also reveal deep aspects of a person's personal theological understanding. The statement 'I feel I am being punished because of ... ' may grow out of implicit beliefs such as 'Good people do not suffer. I am suffering, therefore I am not good'. In trying to fit the experience of caring for a dying child into a personal theological perspective, the whole question of God's love can be very problematic, as can the idea of God as protector or the answerer of prayer. Key assumptions that help to underpin a person's life are suddenly thrown into question – questioning that in itself can occasion further guilt. In such discussion it is important that we convey an acceptance to the person so that they can begin, in whatever way is helpful for them, to say the unsayable.

Imaginative entering into another person's internal world is not simply the domain of the psychotherapist. It is something we do much of the time for communication to occur at all. In the setting of caring for someone facing a major threat to their basic assumptions, it is vitally important because it is a way of helping them to articulate their fears and break out of a sense of isolation. However, such exploration may not be helpful for everyone and should not be viewed as a compulsory 'technique'. Neither should we press further than the person is prepared to go.

Over time, remembering word pictures is a way of gauging what is happening in a person's inner world. When the heart seems no longer to be stony, but is perhaps felt to be bleeding, then change has occurred and there is a way of talking about what has happened that is mutually meaningful. Or when the picture of God changes from a punishing father to a supportive friend, again there is internal movement and reconstruction.

The process of internal change and reconstruction is hard and long. As carers we can attempt to short-circuit the process because we feel more comfortable. For example, if a person describes a sense of being in a dark hole with no one to care, an immediate response can be: 'It is OK, I care.' Such a statement may be true for the carer, but may not be felt to be true for the person in crisis. They feel in the hole, and they feel alone despite the fact that they are talking to the carer. It is more isolating for them to have their sense of aloneness invalidated and unheard. More helpfully, time could be spent asking what the dark hole is like – how deep is it, are there ways out? This takes the experience seriously and builds a bridge between the worlds of speaker and hearer. In the longer term, it is this that reduces the sense of isolation, rather than words of reassurance. Likewise, in more obviously religious conversations, the statement 'God does not care' can be too easily answered in doctrinal terms such as 'Yes he does, God is love', rather than allowing the person to explore in what way they feel God to be uncaring. In this way, feelings such as anger or rejection can be expressed, rather than hidden.

For the carer, daring to stay with a person as they explore such times of darkness and pain can be daunting and threatening because it can lead the carer to re-evaluate their own assumptions about life's purpose.

Word pictures are by no means the only way through which we can enter imaginatively into the world of another person. They reveal much of themselves through their hobbies, interests, what they watch on video, their musical taste, and the way they talk about these experiences. With children, the toys they like and how they play is also a crucial point of contact. As carers, we should be attentive to all these areas of self-disclosure as they can provide a way for the person to share with us what they may be thinking or feeling at the time. Even if the latest video game is not necessarily going to reveal the depths of another's psyche, our willingness to play conveys much about our interest and respect for the person, which builds trust.

Yet paying attention to these areas in a person's life can reveal deep yearnings and concerns. For example, for someone profoundly physically handicapped, an interest in planes may show a deep yearning for freedom that can be explored with the carer. A great fondness for the films of Arnold Schwarzenegger may reveal a sense of frustration at their own powerlessness. Sharing in drawing or painting, going for outings, are also opportunities for sensing what is of concern – what in their lives seems to be life-giving and what is life-denying. Meaning is personal, though containing interpersonal dimensions as well. We cannot assume we know what a particular symbol or picture will mean to a particular person. We need to explore it in a way that enables them to correct us so that we can understand more fully. Neither should we assume that everyone will express themselves in the same way. For example, men often find articulating feelings difficult and can be easily ignored as they go to 'do' things such as fix the car engine or something equally practical. Important links can be made just talking about engines, in the context of which other things may surface.

I have not distinguished the approach to other members of the family as the issues are similar. According to their age, ability and temperament, each of them is having to discover a new sense of meaning, a new frame of reference, within which to live their lives.

LETTING GO: DYING AND BEREAVEMENT

The process of discovering meaning in the face of the death of a loved child may involve the discussion of what death and dying involves. This can be conducted at a number of levels. Real fear can surround issues such as the possibility of pain, of being alone, of what will happen in a medical sense. Talking through these very practical things with the family in ways that each member can understand is crucial to relieve hidden fears and concerns. People can also have ways of understanding death in a metaphysical sense that can either help or hinder the process of dying when the time comes. If the opportunity arises, it is important to talk through these ideas. The child who is ill may feel unable to talk about things like this with his parents for fear of upsetting them. Parents may not talk with each other or with brothers and sisters. By trying so hard not to hurt each others' feelings a conspiracy of silence is built up that can be isolating and frightening. By building up committed, caring and attentive relationships with family members, we can help to provide a safe forum where such discussion takes place. It may not be with the family as a whole, and may not happen when we think it ought to, but we should provide the space where it becomes possible. Again, with children, play or films can provide an arena where such discussion can happen.

If the talk or play is of war, the question 'I wonder what happens to all the ones who get shot?' may elicit the reaction 'They are taken to hospital' or a discussion of personal constructs around the experience of death. Such metaphysical constructs are important because they can reveal deep fears about death and the after-life. 'Only good boys go to heaven' can be a remark made to a small, well child that later on as a teenager, facing both a mixed up past and the imminence of death, creates great fear of what the after-life may be like. 'Jesus

takes the good ones to be stars' can be well meaning, but could lead
a younger sibling to try to be as bad as possible because Jesus may
come for him too! If the person has little concept of an after-life they
may be comfortable with the idea of death as pain-free sleep – but
for a sibling who cannot quite understand, such a notion of sleep may
be deeply distressing. Likewise, what happens to the body – burial
or cremation – may be important because of certain fears the child
may have about worms or fire. Talking through these areas can be
very painful, but it is important so that when the terminal stage comes
some of the fears have been allayed, practical arrangements made in
terms perhaps of pain control, and a language for talking about what
is going to happen has been developed. For example, if a child strongly
believes in a particular picture of heaven, or a notion such as that a
beloved relative will come to meet him at death, it can be helpful if
he becomes fretful in the terminal stages to talk soothingly about his
own vision of what the after-life may be like.

Part of the preparation for dying can also include symbolic acts of
preparation or the planning of the funeral. If there are particular prized
possessions, it may be important that they are handed on as a way
of caring for the people who are left. Or it may be that the continued
care of something, perhaps a stamp collection or set of models, may
be a way of ensuring that the child will feel remembered. Similarly,
the opportunity literally to say goodbye or to put things right within
particular families can be as important to some children as it is for
adults.*

They may also want a funeral that reflects the sense they have made
out of their illness in terms of readings or choice of hymns and music.
Again, such discussion need not be with the religious minister, though
it is important that whoever is conducting the service is aware of these
requests.

Other members of the family also need to be supported through
this time. The needs of parents are perhaps most clear. They need
to have the space and support to decide how they want this part of
their child's life to be lived. Yet there must also be respect for the time
when they may feel they can no longer stay in the room, and help
for them to return to their child if they are finding this increasingly
difficult and painful. The needs of siblings at this time can often be
overlooked, but their future memories of the experience will be
affected by how they are involved in this stage of terminal care. It
is wise to encourage involvement in natural ways without forcing them
to do things that frighten them. If time has been given to getting to
know their ways of making sense of what is happening, this can be

---

* For a description of work with a child with a terminal illness see Judd [9]. This also
contains a useful bibliography.

made easier. Involvement may range from asking them to bring in a favourite toy to holding hands. It must be remembered that siblings, too, need space and time to play; staff involvement in this in the case of residential care, or the support of a friend or relative at home, can relieve the pressure from the parents.

The moment of death itself may evoke a whole range of feelings. Members of the family will express themselves differently. There is no right way, only their way. Time should be given to the period after death so that goodbyes can be said. The process of preparing the body after death, the choice of clothes and where the body will rest are crucial parts of this process. They can say so much about how the death is understood. Dressing the child in a tracksuit may be an acknowledgement of a sense of the freedom they now experience that they never knew during their earthly life. The words spoken at this time by all members of the family are precious.

Events at the time of death can also be powerfully symbolic and evoke a sense of hope. The appearance of a bright star in the sky, a plane flying overhead, the presence of two magpies, can be deeply reassuring. They are also deeply spiritual because they convey profound meanings about death.

There is a risk that after death people can act as if, in some way, it is all over. The intensity of the moment has gone and for some professionals their involvement will be over. Yet as the literature on bereavement suggests, this is far from the end for the remaining family members. The pain goes on for each of them and this is where follow-up is so important. It continues to enable them each to make sense of what has happened and come to terms with it.

THE FUNERAL

Religous traditions vary in terms of how the body should be treated after death and the timing of funerals. It is important that these are discussed clearly with the family beforehand to ensure that taboos are not broken and further pain caused that can be avoided.* For most people dying in the United Kingdom, the arrangements will be for a broadly Christian funeral. The following remarks will be addressed specifically to that context, but may be relevant to other traditions as well.

The keynote for the funeral is that it must be right for the family, express their love of the child who has died, and that it speaks of their perspective on death. In cases where the child has had strong feelings about the funeral, these may be woven into the service. The family

---

* Useful books include those by Neuberger [10] and Kramer [11].

needs to feel a real sense of freedom to make their own choice of music, hymns and readings, even if there are aspects of the service that are liturgically 'given'.* This permission – for example, to use pop music, a film theme or nursery rhyme – may need to be explicit – 'Did their child have a particular favourite piece of music or Bible story?' 'Do they have songs that mean a lot to them?', and so on. There may need to be a number of meetings to plan the funeral and a lot of help in choosing material. However, it is an important time because it gives a chance for the family to talk through what has happened and to ensure that when they look back on the service they will find in it sources of hope and strength: a sense of things 'being done right'.

This process can be complicated because people may change their minds or find it hard to say what they mean. There may also be past experience of funerals that can affect how they approach this one. Liaison between the minister and undertaker, so that the service is not rushed forward until things are clearer to the family, can be crucial. This also gives time for the family to decide if they want anything placed in the coffin with their child. Related to this is the choice of flowers as expressions of love and of the personality of the child. If a parent is too upset to go to the florist alone, someone who knows their wishes should go with them so that the colours and design are appropriate. Flowers can also be a way of involving other children in the family, for example helping them to sign flower cards and choose designs. In a profound sense, the funeral is a family affair.

The funeral address itself is also important. In considering the words used, thought needs to be given to the way in which the child and the family make sense of death. The pictures in words that they use can be a starting point for an appreciation of the child's life and ultimate destiny. Particular events and memories can have profound significance at this point. For example, a child who enjoyed travelling suggests the analogy of a 'journey'. A child with multiple handicaps may have had a particular physical or emotional characteristic deeply valued by the family – their eyes or their smile may have been the means through which the family glimpsed the character of their child. At this stage the value of listening carefully to how members of the family have made sense of the illness is vital so that this can be married to the understanding of death in a given religious tradition. A sermon that does not seek to integrate personal understanding

---

* Useful approaches to the conduct of children's funerals are found in the 'Order of Christian Funerals' prepared by the Roman Catholic Church published by Geoffrey Chapman, London, 1990. Some material is also given in the Alternative Service Book, Hodder and Stoughton, London, 1980. For deaths in infancy and early childhood a very useful booklet is available from the Church of Scotland called 'Pastoral Guidelines and a Funeral Service for Stillbirths and Deaths in Early Infancy', Oxford University Press, Oxford, 1986.

with religious understanding, but concentrates largely on the latter, runs the risk of failing to meet the family in their need.

The funeral may have been the first point of contact between a family and a religious minister. The period after the funeral can be especially valuable for a family to explore the meaning of their child's death within an explicitly religious framework. Because the family will probably be having to rediscover a more regular pattern of life after possible years of an erratic lifestyle, they may take quite a long time to begin to grieve. This means that follow-up after the funeral may have to be over quite a long period and not simply discontinued when things seem more settled. Some Martin House families describe the second year as being more traumatic than the first.

RELIGIOUS ACTS AND THEIR PLACE IN CARE

For most of this chapter the emphasis has been on spiritual care seen in the broad sense as being concerned with helping the family in their quest to give meaning to the events surrounding their child's illness. Clearly religious beliefs are an important aspect of this. In addition to beliefs, the symbolic rituals associated with specific faiths can be very powerful expressions of what a family may wish to celebrate about the life of their child. As the Anglican chaplain at Martin House I was privileged to share in a number of Christian rituals with families who came to stay. My very personal reflections will form the basis of the following discussion. I hope some of the points raised will have relevance to those who are ministers of other faiths as they seek to provide spiritual care.

The keynote of religious care for a family as it finds expression in religious acts is the attempt to bring together the traditional meaning of the ritual and the particular meanings the family bring to the event. This does not necessarily mean changing the ritual unrecognizably; rather it means making it personal. At one level this can involve using the familiar names of the child and the family members. Ideally, though, it should mean that either through a prayer, a reading or a symbolic act the particular meanings that the family bring to the experience are explicitly recognized and honoured.

Baptism

Occasionally a family would seek baptism in the Martin House chapel which was performed with the consent of their local clergy. Such baptisms were not strictly emergencies. Rather they were important acts embarked upon in the knowledge that their child had a life-threatening condition. The format of the Anglican baptism service contains clear assumptions about the child coming in later years to confirmation. Clearly for many of the children using Martin House this was an unrealistic hope, and if included insensitively in the service could have been upsetting for parents.

In talking with parents, the things they wanted to celebrate through baptism were the uniqueness of their child, the fact that they are loved by God and would ultimately be safe with him in heaven, the sense of being a family bound together in the care of their ill child, and the continued need for God's support as they moved into an uncertain future.

Clearly many of these ideas are already implicit in the baptism service, but its language can seem to people unfamiliar with it to be rather clumsy in its expression of these truths. With the permission of the Archbishop of York, we experimented with ways of celebrating the baptism service that were both true to traditional understandings of baptism as rebirth, cleaning and incorporation into the body of Christ; yet at the same time sought through prayers and symbolic acts to draw in more explicitly the concerns of the family.

Hence, more was made of the actual naming of the child as an expression of their uniqueness. The naming was accompanied by the laying of the priest's hand on the child and prayer. The exorcism was transformed into an assurance that the child's name was written in the book of life, rather than the more theologically complex words which are about being led in the light and obedience of Christ [12]. The signing of the cross was made much of as a way of talking about the child sharing in the new life celebrated at Easter. It is also a way of talking of God's light in the darkness and uncertainty of the future both for the child himself and for the rest of the family. Giving candles to all family members, which are not actual baptismal candles, can be a powerful sign both of solidarity and future hope. The final prayers may also be elaborated upon to speak to the particular needs of the family.

These have been the ideas we pursued. They are offered as ideas rather than hard and fast rules. Clearly the context of baptism in Martin House chapel is very different from that in a Sunday service at a parish church where the greater concern may be to establish the solidarity of the sick child with that of the other children being baptized.

However, whether the baptism is done as an emergency or in the context described, it is crucial that the articles left with the family such as the baptism certificate, the baptismal candle, and the Bible are inscribed with the child's name and the date with great care. They will become an important link with the child and with the experience of baptism that was celebrated.

Holy Communion

As a rule, the Anglican practice is to admit to communion after confirmation. In the context of Martin House chapel the celebration of Holy Communion became an important time of solidarity for all present, which meant that excluding some from communicating seemed in opposition to the inclusive ethos of the house. The symbolism of communion itself – offering, breaking, sharing – and the drama of resurrection following crucifixion can be very powerful in the context of hospice care. The book *Celebration* by Margaret Spufford movingly describes this [13].

One communion service each week was very much celebrated with the children in mind using a simplified liturgy and encouraging them to choose the theme of the service, pick appropriate readings and compose prayers. It was a moving experience to be a part of a liturgy that expressed the children's own struggling to understand their illness in the context of the world's suffering. For example, some of the boys with muscular dystrophy felt close to people held as hostage or as prisoners of conscience. They recognized the sense of being deprived of freedom. The liturgy provided them with the opportunity to give form to the profound sense of empathy they felt with such prisoners. Although such an approach to liturgy is more easily possible in a residential context, a parish congregation would be enriched if a sick child was encouraged to articulate something of his own understanding of illness as part of Sunday worship. It is one way in which the child can feel that he is offering a real contribution to the life of the church that neither marginalizes him nor makes him feel only the powerless recipient of care.

Some children with severe handicaps may be very limited in the liturgical involvement they can make, yet the use of music with shakers and rattles can enable them to make a real and valued contribution.

Laying on of hands/annointing

As noted already, the use of the ministry to the sick needs to be handled with great care. While prayer for healing may be entirely appropriate, its meaning must be made clear. For many families, even after a diagnosis of a terminal condition there is a deep desire to prove the doctors wrong. Denial and searching are clearly documented parts of the process of adapting to change. The ministry to the sick must not become a means of denial that stops the family as a whole coming to terms with the pain of their situation and beginning to face the likely outcome. It is also important that they do not feel unfaithful or guilty if the child dies. However, this ministry can be a great help as a sign of God's involvement in the situation and His continued care, in spite of what they may feel to be all appearances to the contrary.

Annointing with oil can also be a great comfort as a sign of God's presence and of a commending of the child into His care.

It is crucial, however, that if called to administer any form of sacramental care that this is seen as an act of love, not something mechanical. Time should be taken in preparing the family and in visiting afterwards to ensure that the sacramental act is given a context and is not simply a 'one off'.

Memorial services

This is a form of service that is relevant more to forms of residential care. At Martin House, as at Helen House, we hold yearly memorial services. They attempt to help the families in their journey of bereavement, by acknowledging the pain as well as the hidden hope that is also present. Hence the choice of hymns and readings reflects both pain and hope. The service sheets reflect this in their use of the rainbow and butterfly as symbols of hope. Symbols are also used in the service. Candles and flower bulbs are two examples. The bulbs have been particularly valued as they are a practical outworking of the mystery of death and new life.*

WE HURT TOO

Spiritual care is personally involving. It can be no other because it is dealing with the sense we make of life and death. In some way each of us has to address these questions. Particular children or family dynamics can evoke strong reactions in us. They may trigger past hurts, or highlight an area of our present life that is unresolved.

It is crucial that we have people with whom we can talk so that we may address our own personal feelings. The risk of not doing so is that we address them through our involvement with the family. This means that we cannot simply accompany them on the journey, but rather try to show them which way to go, in accordance with our own perspectives and needs.

Such personal care for ourselves should not wait until we feel we need it, but should be part of our ongoing work. At Martin House a staff support group meets weekly with an outside facilitator to

---

* If this is something you have to arrange and would like more details, please write direct to Martin House. The address is given in the list of resources at the end of the book.

allow feelings among the care team to be aired and personal issues addressed. Part of its value lies in the discovery that experiences that staff members felt to be idiosyncratic responses to the pains and joys of such care were actually shared with others. There could then be a real sense that others knew how they felt, thus overcoming the sense of isolation that such work can bring. It also permits the expression of feelings that as 'carers' are hard to acknowledge, such as frustration and anger towards those in care. For some people a group situation is not helpful and provision was therefore made for people to meet one to one to discuss their feelings.

The chaplain, as a figure both inside and outside the institution, has a key role in such support. The above discussion on the use of imagery and the linking of past and present hurts is as relevant to staff seeking to 'make sense' as it is to the care of families. The need for such support for those involved in community care or in hospital can be overlooked but is very necessary.

There can, however, be times when we should be particularly aware of the need for such support. If we have had a major loss in the recent past, through bereavement, divorce, a child leaving home, or whatever, we are more vulnerable to issues concerned with loss. Likewise, if we notice, or others notice in us, short temperedness, feelings of anger, a tendency to tears, problems relaxing, and so on then we are perhaps tired and in need of both rest and a chance to address our own needs. To go through such times is not to fail, it is to be honestly human.

CONCLUSION

This chapter has attempted to raise issues in spiritual care that are of general concern. There is no one way of 'doing' spiritual care. We each vary as people, as do the families with whom we work. To a large extent this chapter articulates a perspective on spiritual care that has grown out of the experience of residential care at Martin House. It seems to be relevant to other contexts as well. In simple terms, it is about trying to be alongside people, helping them to know you are there and that you are not afraid of some of the feelings that they may have, giving them the time and space to address their hopes and fears in a meaningful way, whatever their age. In this way they can begin to make sense of a situation that, at first sight, can seem utterly senseless. Such care is both costly at a personal level and a great privilege, and is in no way the exclusive territory of 'religious people'.

ACKNOWLEDGEMENTS

Thank you to the staff and families of Martin House who helped to teach me what it meant to be a priest. For his support and interest, thanks to Revd Richard Seed, fellow chaplain and friend. For proof reading and advice, thanks to the Venerable Hugh Buckingham and Chris Kavanagh. For helping me to listen to pictures, thanks to Dr Miller-Mair and the Crichton Royal psychologists.

REFERENCES

1. Sarnoff-Schiff, H. (1979) *The Bereaved Parent*, Souvenir Press, London.
2. Campbell, A. (1986) *Rediscovering Pastoral Care*, Darton Longman and Todd, London, p. 16.
3. Cassidy, S. (1988) *Sharing the Darkness*, Darton Longman and Todd, London, p. 63.
4. Adams, D. (1979) *The Hitch-hiker's Guide to the Galaxy*, Pan, London.
5. *The Spiritual Exercises of St Ignatius* (1978) (trans. D. Fleming) Institute of Jesuit Studies, St Louis, Mo.
6. Eliot, T.S. (1986) 'Burnt Norton', in *Collected Poems 1909–1962*, Faber and Faber, London.
7. Miller-Mair, J. (1989) *Between Psychology and Psychotherapy – a Poetics of Experience*, Routledge, London.
8. Rowe, D. (1989) *The Construction of Life and Death*, Fontana, London.
9. Judd, D. (1989) *Give Sorrow Words*, Free Association Books. London.
10. Neuberger, J. (1990) *Caring for Dying People of Differing Faiths*, The Kisa Sainsbury Foundation, Austen Cornish, London.
11. Kramer, K. (1988) *The Sacred Art of Dying*, Paulist Press, New York.
12. Alternative Service Book (1980) Hodder and Stoughton, London, pp. 243–9.
13. Spufford, M. (1989) *Celebration*, Fountain Press, London.

CHAPTER 9

Symptom control in dying children

Michael Brady

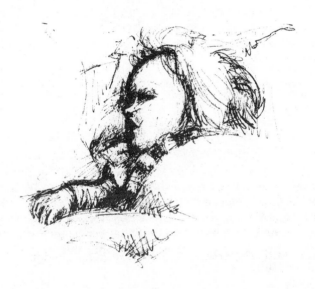

Death in childhood is, thankfully, a rare event. Sometimes there is little or no warning, as in accidental death. At other times death will follow a prolonged illness which will ultimately enter a terminal phase. This stage is characterized by the cessation of active or aggressive treatment and the acceptance of the inevitability of death. Treatment is no longer aimed at cure, nor necessarily prolonging life, but rather at alleviating symptoms and providing support for the child and family. Although the goals of treatment may have changed they are no less worthy nor demanding and require as much care and consideration as the preceding active phase of treatment.

Because death from chronic illness in childhood is a relatively uncommon event – there were some 1171 such deaths in England and Wales in 1981 – few health professionals will gain extensive experience in providing paediatric terminal care. On average, a British general practitioner is likely to be involved in one or two cases in an entire career. Not surprisingly, therefore, it can be a daunting prospect. The attending physician may be faced with a child dying from a rare illness of which he has no previous experience. Fear on the part of the carers can therefore be a significant barrier to the provision of effective terminal care.

This should not be the case, however, as many of the principles of symptom control in dying children are identical to those in adults. Carers can therefore draw on their experience of adult terminal care. Furthermore, extensive knowledge of rare diseases is not of prime importance in planning symptom control. The vast array of disease processes in fact presents a relatively small number of therapeutic problems. Finally, with a few exceptions, children are no more prone to side-effects of drugs prescribed in appropriate doses than adults. Undue fear of side-effects should not, therefore, be allowed to preclude necessary treatment.

GENERAL PRINCIPLES OF SYMPTOM CONTROL

The setting for terminal care

Much has been written about the most appropriate setting for the provision of terminal care. Many feel that this is best provided in the family home if this is the wish of the child and his family. Sometimes circumstances or preference dictate that care be undertaken elsewhere, in a familiar hospital unit or perhaps a hospice. Although most of the following comments are based on personal experience in a children's hospice, this approach to care is equally applicable to the hospital or community setting.

The importance of a team approach

No single person will possess all the attributes and abilities needed in the course of the final illness. Each member of the team will contribute their own personal and professional skills. Team members provide mutual emotional support for one another as well as for the family.

Good communication between team members is essential. All must be aware of the problems faced and their proposed management. A cohesive strategy and unified approach is needed as conflicting information or advice merely leads to confusion and mistrust.

The approach to symptoms

As with adults, symptoms are rarely simple physical events but, more often, complex experiences with physical, emotional, social and spiritual components. Though these may be more difficult to recognize in children, all must be considered if treatment is to be successful. Remember, too, that the child's suffering is shared by his family. Their pain must be acknowledged and appropriate support offered.

SPECIAL CONSIDERATIONS IN CHILDREN

The heterogeneity of children

Children differ from adults in that they are growing and developing. Their physical, intellectual and social abilities are constantly changing. Assessment and management must be geared to children's differing stages of development.

The nature of terminal illness in children

Terminal illnesses in childhood are far less numerous but far more varied than those seen in adults, where neoplastic disease predominates. In some cases, such as childhood leukaemia, the terminal stage of the illness follows soon after the cessation of active treatment and pursues a relentless and fairly predictable downhill course. In others, such as metabolic or neurodegenerative disease, the course of the illness is longer and less predictable. A period of rapid deterioration, when it seems that life expectancy is measured in hours or days, may be followed by a plateau where the child's condition stabilizes for weeks or even months. This makes recognition of the terminal stage of the illness extremely difficult and places enormous strain on the family. They have put all their emotional and physical resources into what are believed to be the last days of their child's life only to find that the seemingly inevitable does not occur. The agonizing process may be repeated several times before death eventually ensues.

COMMUNICATION PROBLEMS

Assessment of symptoms usually relies heavily on verbal information offered by the patient. In children this may be lacking for various reasons. Young children may lack the vocabulary required to describe the symptoms or may simply be shy and reserved with adults. In other cases communication is impaired by profound mental handicap such as that seen in many progressive central nervous system disorders. It is interesting to note that the recorded incidence of some symptoms is lower in non-communicating than communicating children. Although this may in part reflect a genuine difference in the incidence of symptoms in the two groups, it may also be that symptoms are not recognized where communication is lacking.

Thus, we must often rely on our own observations and those of parents and other carers who are familiar with the child. They may recognize patterns of vocalization, facial expression, posture and movement which suggest the presence of pain or other symptoms. Take their comments seriously – they are usually right.

The need for parental involvement

We often rely on a child's parents for information essential to management. Children usually look first to their parents for information and support, perhaps to a trusted nurse second and usually the doctor last. Parents are often required to take decisions regarding treatment on behalf of their child. They will be suffering alongside him.

For these and many other reasons close parental involvement and cooperation are essential. The purpose of any treatment prescribed and the way in which it should be administered should be explained carefully. Parents should be encouraged to be involved in day-to-day care not left feeling helpless by professionals who 'take over' their child. The satisfaction of having coped with difficulty and provided the best possible care for their child is often a source of comfort to parents when bereavement finally comes.

Parental perceptions of symptoms need to be explored and their fears discussed. Some symptoms, for example, noisy breathing, may not trouble the dying child but may be deeply distressing to the parents. Parents may have unwarranted concerns which, if identified, should be allayed by appropriate reassurance.

Drug administration in children

Specific drugs will be discussed in more detail in the sections which follow. However, a few general points are worthy of mention.

Children do not like injections. This is particularly true of wasted children for whom injections will be painful and unpleasant. Always use the oral route when possible. If injections are unavoidable, the subcutaneous route is kinder. If repeated injections are envisaged a continuous subcutaneous infusion should be considered. Some children may have established venous access, such as a Hickman line, and this presents a useful alternative route of administration. Others may have a nasogastric tube which may be employed to administer syrups, suspensions and crushed or soluble tablets. Rectal administration is useful for some drugs but remember to prescribe suppositories of appropriate size. Sublingual administration is only practical in older children and is of limited value.

When giving drugs orally, bear in mind that children often prefer tablets or capsules to syrups which are often sickly sweet. Soluble tablets or solutions may be flavoured with cordial or fizzy drinks according to the child's preference. Where the child is unable to take tablets but no syrup or solution is commonly available it is worth having a word with the pharmacist as it may be possible to prepare a suspension, though stability may be a problem. Alternatively, crushed tablets or the contents of capsules may be mixed into ice cream, yoghurt or some other favourite food.

PAIN

Of all the symptoms we are asked to treat, pain is the most common and the most feared. Parents dread their children suffering severe pain above all else. The pain in terminal illness, particularly in malignant disease, is typically chronic, constant and without meaning. It serves no useful purpose and slowly erodes the morale of both child and parent.

The physiology of pain

It is important to realize that pain is not a simple physiological event but rather a complex experience with physical, psychological, social and spiritual components – all of which contribute to what has been termed 'total pain'. The psychosocial and spiritual factors contributing to pain, and indeed other symptoms, are considered elsewhere. The following is merely a summary of the anatomical and physiological basis of pain perception. There are broadly two clinically significant types of pain – nociceptive pain and deafferentation pain.

Nociceptive pain

Here a painful stimulus gives rise to an electrical impulse in an afferent (sensory) neuron which is transmitted to the sensory area of the parietal cortex as shown in Figure 9.1. This is a simplified representation of a fairly complex event. The transmission of impulses is a combined electrical and chemical process allowing conduction along neurons and transfer from neuron to neuron across synaptic junctions.

Pain of this type is usually sensitive to opiates which modify transmissions of pain via opiate receptors within the central nervous system.

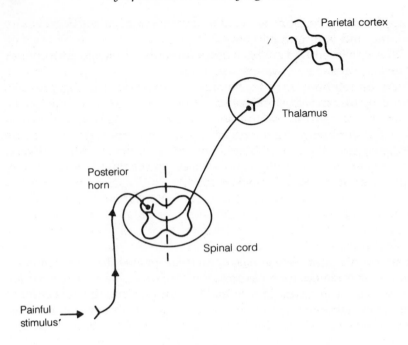

Fig. 9.1 Transmission of nociceptive pain.

Deafferentation pain

Here the normal pathway of nerve conduction is interrupted, for
example by nerve compression or destruction in malignant disease.
This gives rise to a series of anatomical neurochemical and
physiological changes resulting in abnormal pain conduction. The pain
is thus accompanied by altered sensation and is of unusual quality
(stabbing or burning). Pain of this type is typically insensitive to opiates
as there are changes in the opiate receptors with reduction of their
numbers, alteration of their site and malfunction of remaining
receptors.

Pain is further modified within the CNS by complex enhancing/
inhibiting systems which perhaps explain the wide variation in pain
perception and allow for integration of cognitive/emotional factors.
These systems are not fully understood but the 'gate control' theory
encompasses a number of components which may modify pain
perception.

Assessment of pain

In adult terminal care it is desirable and usually possible to arrive at
an accurate diagnosis of the cause of pain and an accurate assessment

of its severity. Often this will not be possible in children. Rarely, for example, will young children be able to give an elaborate account of the site and quality of pain; 'it hurts' may be the only information obtained.

In assessing pain three areas must be examined – is pain present, if so how severe is it, and finally what is its cause?

Is pain present?

The presence of pain is obvious when the information is volunteered. Often, however, it will not be. This may be because of the communication barriers imposed by lack of vocabulary, for example in infants and in children with mental handicap. Sometimes even communicative children will deny pain, though their silence and misery speak volumes. A child's denial of pain may simply result from a stoical attitude or from a desire to protect his parents from suffering. Alternatively if previous admission to pain has led to an injection, the child may be reluctant to do so again for fear of the consequences.

In the absence of a verbal complaint of pain one must rely on nonverbal clues. In infants, facial expression, posture, body movements and the quality of the cry may suggest pain. Typically the eyes are open, the corners of the mouth downwards and outwards, and the platysma contracted. The cry is often loud and of abnormal quality. In older children insomnia, loss of appetite, irritability and disinterest in play are useful features to look for. These clues may only be gleaned by spending some time observing the child. The comments of parents or care staff who know the child well are invaluable and usually accurate. If in doubt as to whether pain is present, bear in mind that 80% of children will have pain in advanced life-threatening illness. Prescription of analgesics on the balance of probabilities, at least as a therapeutic trial, therefore seems reasonable.

How severe is the pain?

Assessment of severity may be made by either informal observation or by formal measurement. Usually a combination is employed.

Informal observation may provide the only information available in young and non-communicative children. In older children it may provide useful additional information. Watching a child while in his room or socializing with other children may yield evidence of pain denied or minimized by the child when formally questioned. Pain may be given away by grimaces, protective movements of painful limbs or simple reluctance to play with other children. These observations may provide a more accurate indication of the severity of pain than the brave 'not too bad' offered to the parent or doctor.

Where possible **formal objective measurement** of pain is desirable in planning pain management and assessing the effectiveness of treatment. Most systems have been developed primarily for use in adults and, because of the factors outlined above, their use in children is limited. Older children may be able to produce reliable information from standard adult pain assessment scales such as the visual analogue scale (VAS) or intensity rating scale (IRS). Pain maps, such as that produced by the King's College Pain Relief Unit, may also be helpful. The site of pain is marked and descriptions of the pain noted alongside. Repeated scale ratings may provide objective assessment of effectiveness of treatment.

Younger children are more difficult to assess and soon tire of formal testing. The Elland Colour Tool is one system devised for use in younger children. The child is asked to colour areas on an outline on the assessment chart, indicating the areas where they feel pain. Several colours are selected by the child, each corresponding to different severity of pain. Any comments made by the child may be added alongside.

What is the cause of the pain?

It is important, though not always possible, to arrive at an accurate diagnosis of the cause of pain. The cause of pain will in large measure determine its treatment. Bear in mind that often more than one pain is present and each individual pain may have several different components.

From a therapeutic point of view pain may be divided into three categories:

(a) Opiate sensitive pain;
(b) Opiate resistant pain;
(c) Opiate 'irrelevant' pain.

Opiate sensitive pain

Most pain from direct visceral involvement, i.e. from abdominal, pelvic and intrathoracic organs, falls into this category. Typically the pain is a continous dull ache though it may be sharp if the organ moves with change in position. It responds well to treatment with opiates alone in most instances.

Two types of visceral pain are perhaps worthy of specific mention. **Colic** is common and in children usually related to constipation rather than obstruction, which is rare. The pain will be reduced by prescription of opiates but they will of course merely exacerbate the situation. Always look for a loaded colon or full rectum in any child with abdominal pain. **Gastric irritation** is most commonly seen in children prescribed non-steroidal anti-inflammatories (NSAIDs) or steroids. If possible the causative agent should be stopped. If this is not possible, symptoms may be relieved by prescription of an H_2 blocker.

Opiate resistant pain

Sometimes pain is either partially or completely resistant to opiate analgesics. In the former, adjuvant treatment with co-analgesic drugs or other therapy will be needed to augment the partial response to opiates. In the latter, opiates will not help even in large doses and alternative, appropriate treatment should be instituted.

(i) Partial opiate resistance Bone pain, pain due to soft tissue infiltration, pain due to nerve compression and headache from raised intracranial pressure (ICP) are only partially sensitive to opiates.

Bone pain is typically dull aching pain made worse by movement. Rapidly increasing pain on movement suggests an impending pathological fracture. Bone tenderness is usually present. The diagnosis may be confirmed by X-ray but a bone scan is more accurate.

Palliative radiotherapy is the treatment of choice for isolated bone secondaries. As well as providing excellent pain relief it may prevent pathological fracture.

NSAIDs are also helpful – particularly where multiple secondaries are present. They inhibit the synthesis of prostaglandins which mediate bone pain and osteolysis. Corticosteroids, which also inhibit prostaglandin synthesis, are an alternative.

In **soft tissue infiltration** NSAIDs and corticosteroids may again be helpful. If infection is present topical antiseptic measures, debridement and antibiotics by mouth may be helpful. Metronidazole often helps to reduce the unpleasant smell associated with sloughing malignant ulceration. Topical anaesthetics may help but there is a risk of local sensitivity reaction.

The pain of **nerve compression** is typically associated with numbness and corresponds to one or more nerve territories. There may be signs of altered sensory, and possibly motor, function. Corticosteroids will reduce tumour-associated oedema which is often a significant component of nerve compression. Initial high doses are reduced after seven days.

Raised intracranial pressure produces headache which is severe, diffuse and often exacerbated by stooping or bending. There may be associated blurred vision and vomiting. Papilloedema may be present. It is most commonly seen in children with cerebral tumours. Corticosteroids are usually helpful, again because they reduce tumour-associated oedema. As in nerve compression, initial high doses should be reduced after seven days.

Raised ICP may also be seen in infants with hydrocephalus where, because of poor prognosis, a shunt has not been fitted or where a blocked shunt is not to be replaced. The infant is irritable and vomits. The neck may be retracted and the fontanelle bulging. A high pitched 'cerebral' cry may be present. Temporary relief may be obtained by performing a ventricular tap if the fontanelle is patent.

(ii) Complete opiate resistance Pain due to muscle spasm and to nerve infiltration/destruction is usually insensitive to opiates.

Muscle spasm is common in paediatric terminal care. It is most commonly seen in neurological disease where spastic paresis is present. It may also be seen as a secondary phenomenon in primary and secondary bone tumours or where there is skeletal deformity. It is often difficult to relieve and is distressing for the child and parents. Spasm may be severe and unpredictable. Analgesics are unhelpful and the parents are unable to hold or nurse their distressed, rigid child.

Muscle relaxants such as baclofen or diazepam are usually helpful (see p. 158). Instruction of family and carers regarding handling and positioning is equally important. The advice of an experienced paediatric physiotherapist is invaluable.

Nerve destruction/infiltration gives rise to the characteristic deafferentation pain described above. The pain is usually dermatomal and may be increased by lightly touching the skin in the affected area. It may be described as burning or stabbing. Burning pain may respond to antidepressant treatment. Stabbing pain may respond to anticonvulsants such as carbamazepine or sodium valproate. If there is associated nerve compression corticosteroids may be helpful. Often the pain will be resistant to all drug measures and a nerve block may be required.

Opiate irrelevant pain

This description has been applied to pain whose principal components are spiritual, psychological and social rather than physical. It is less easily recognized in children than adults. The child who is in pain because he is frightened of dying or because he sees his exhausted parents daily suffering will not be helped by an analgesic. He does not need a drug but the opportunity to discuss his fears and anxieties. His emotional and spiritual needs must be addressed. His family must be given support and the time to discuss their feelings. Sadly, it is often easier to give a prescription than to give of ourselves.

GENERAL PRINCIPLES OF PAIN CONTROL

Look for pain

As discussed previously pain may not be volunteered and by the time it is eventually presented may be long established and consequently more difficult to treat. The presence of pain should therefore be actively sought.

Diagnose the cause

Where possible the cause of pain should be determined, but this can be difficult in children. Often the cause must initially be presumed on the basis of probabilities, guided by knowledge of the pathological process involved in the underlying disease, and the response to previous analgesics. Thus a child in pain with a neurological disease where muscle spasticity is present and where the pain has not responded to weak opioids is likely to benefit from a muscle relaxant rather than a prescription for a stronger opioid.

Distinguishing opiate resistant pain is particularly important. Sadly this is often not possible initially and the conclusion is only reached when rapidly increasing opiate doses fail to control pain.

Follow the analgesic staircase

This model of analgesic prescription is well established, with step-wise progression from a non-opioid analgesic to a weak opioid and finally a strong opioid. There are, however, circumstances in which the approach may be modified. For example, in infants under 1 year of age there is a dearth of weak opioids so that direct progression from non-opioid to strong opioid is appropriate. Likewise a child presenting with severe pain at an advanced stage of terminal illness warrants immediate prescription of a strong opioid.

Keep it simple

A host of possible analgesics is available. Familiarity with a few drugs is far·more useful than a sketchy knowledge of many.

Although other drugs will be described in the text, the vast majority of cases can be managed with just one or two drugs from each class.

Use regular doses

Pain in terminal illness is usually continuous. The only role for p.r.n. (i.e. as required) analgesia is for breakthrough pain – its prescription for continuous pain is inadequate. Analgesics should be prescribed as regular doses with a frequency appropriate to the drug involved.

Give drugs orally

Drugs given by injection are no more effective than those given orally. The only indication for injected analgesics is inability to administer drugs orally, perhaps in the comatose patient or where swallowing is impossible owing, for example, to a painful mouth or oesophageal obstruction.

Set goals

Particularly where pain has gone unrecognized or untreated for some time it may prove difficult to achieve adequate pain control quickly. It is important to set goals to achieve in order of priority.

The first goal should be to provide sleep undisturbed by pain. This is almost always attainable and is a significant step forward for the family demoralized by sleepless nights. The second goal is to provide complete relief from pain while at rest. This is usually, though not always, possible. Finally we aim to allow the child to be pain-free on movement or handling. This is by no means always possible.

Re-assess regularly

Adequacy of pain control should be re-assessed regularly and treatment adjusted accordingly.

AVAILABLE ANALGESICS

Analgesics may be conveniently divided into three classes – non-opioids, weak opioids and strong opioids, which are usually prescribed sequentially according to the analgesic staircase.

The most useful drugs are;

Non-opioid: paracetamol.
Weak opioid: codeine (or dihyrocodeine).
Strong opioid: morphine or diamorphine.

Non-opioids

These weak pain killers are suitable for mild pain. Aspirin is a useful drug but because of its association with Reye's syndrome it is now contraindicated in children under 12.

Paracetamol is thus the principal drug in this class. It is well tolerated and toxicity (such as the hepatotoxicity noted in overdose) is rare in therapeutic dosage. It has a useful additional antipyretic action and is available as tablets and soluble tablets (500 mg), an elixir (120 or 250 mg/5 ml) and suppositories (120 or 500 mg).

Doses of non-opioid analgesics

The appropriate doses for the various age groups are set out in Table 9.1.

Table 9.1 Doses of non-opioid analgesics

	Age group				
	0–1	2–5	6–12	13–16	Frequency
Paracetamol	60–120 mg	120–250 mg	250–500 mg	500–1000 mg	4–6 hrly
Aspirin	–	–	–	300–600 mg	6 hrly

Weak opioids

Codeine is the principal drug in this class. It is stronger than aspirin or paracetamol and is safe in long-term use. It may, however, suppress the cough reflex and constipation is common. It is suitable for children over 1 year old in doses of 1–3 mg/kg/24 hours. It is available as tablets (15, 30 and 60 mg), a linctus (3 mg or 15 mg/5 ml) and an injection for i.m. use (60 mg/ml).

Dihydrocodeine is similar in potency to codeine. Again it causes constipation. It is not recommended for children under 4 years old. Thereafter it is given in doses of 2–4 mg/kg/24 hours. It is available as tablets (30 mg), elixir (10 mg/5 ml) and injection for s.c. or i.m. use (50 mg/ml). Modified release tablets are available which may be given every 12 hours (DHC Continus 60 mg m/r).

Codeine is available in a number of compound preparations with paracetamol. Tylex capsules (codeine 30 mg and paracetamol 500 mg) are one example. Co-codamol (codeine 8 mg and paracetamol 500 mg) contain less codeine but are available as soluble tablets. Although the combination of centrally and peripherally acting analgesics seems logical it is doubtful that such compound preparations offer substantial benefits over codeine alone.

Dextropropoxyphene is a poor analgesic when used alone. When combined with paracetamol, e.g. coproxamol (dextropropoxyphene 32.5 mg and paracetamol 325 mg) it is perhaps more effective.

Although a variety of preparations are available within this group, it is generally preferable to use and be familiar with just one or two. If a weak opioid has been prescribed in adequate dosage and pain persists then progress to a strong opioid. Do not be tempted to try other weak opioids in the hope that a strong opioid will be avoided. This usually achieves nothing and merely delays attainment of pain control.

Doses of weak opioid analgesics

The appropriate doses for the various age groups are set out in Table 9.2.

Table 9.2 Doses of weak opioid analgesics

	Age group				
	0–1	2–5	6–12	13–16	Frequency
Codeine	–	10–20 mg	20–30 mg	30–60 mg	4 hrly
Dihydrocodeine	–	–	15–30 mg	30–60 mg	4 hrly
Coproxamol	–	–	1 tab.	1–2 tabs	4–6 hrly)

Strong opioids

The majority of children dying from malignant disease will require strong opioid analgesics at some stage in their illness. In children with non-malignant lethal disease strong opioids are less frequently prescribed and then often for indications other than pain, such as cough or dyspnoea.

Not infrequently, appropriate prescription of a strong opioid is delayed or avoided because of undue fear of side-effects or addiction. Children are in fact no more likely than adults to develop opioid side-effects when drugs are given in appropriate doses, except perhaps in the first month of life when morphine crosses the blood–brain barrier more readily and is metabolized more slowly so that respiratory depression is more likely. Nor will children given adequate, regular doses of strong opioid become addicted. Opioids will not shorten the child's life nor, after the first few days, will they usually produce significant sedation. All these points are worth stressing to the parents before treatment is commenced.

Morphine and diamorphine

Although a number of strong opioids are available, morphine and diamorphine remain the drugs of choice. They are equally effective but their potencies differ, diamorphine being more potent than morphine. Either may be given orally – though only morphine is available in the useful slow release form. If injections are required, diamorphine is preferred as it is more soluble – 1 g dissolves in only 1.6 ml of water. The equivalent doses of oral morphine, oral diamorphine and injected diamorphine are as follows:

Oral morphine = Oral diamorphine = Diamorphine injection
   3 mg   2 mg   1 mg

Thus if a child receiving 30 mg of oral morphine/24 hours is no longer able to tolerate oral medication, 10 mg of diamorphine injection will be required/24 hours.

Morphine may be administered as an oral solution prepared by the pharmacist by dissolving morphine in chloroform water. It is possible to adjust the strength so that the dose volume is convenient, usually 5 ml. Smaller volumes administered from a syringe or graduated pipette may be useful in infants. The solution can be made more palatable by flavouring it with a cordial according to the child's preference. Oramorph is a stable proprietary morphine solution available in concentrations of 10 mg/5 ml or 100 mg/5 ml. Morphine, or diamorphine, tablets are also available (10 mg) but they are not as useful as solutions as the dose is less flexible. Morphine solution should be administered every 4 hours. Giving a double dose at bed time usually avoids the need for a dose in the middle of the night.

Morphine sulphate modified release tablets, MST Continus, offer the advantage of infrequent adminstration. A 12 hourly schedule is generally recommended, though it is often necessary to prescribe MST 8 hourly in younger children to achieve consistent analgesia. MST tablets are available in a useful range of strengths, 5 mg, 10 mg, 30 mg, 60 mg, 100 mg and 200 mg. Contrary to the manufacturer's instructions, the tablets may be crushed without substantially affecting the modified release system. The crushed tablets may be mixed with a favourite food or administered via a nasogastric tube. The recent introduction of MST suspension should provide a simple and more reliable means of administration where tablets cannot be taken. The contents of sachets containing 20 mg or 30 mg of slow release morphine sulphate are mixed with 10 ml of water prior to administration. Because of its modified release formulation, MST Continus has a slow onset of action and is therefore inappropriate for breakthrough pain.

Assuming that the child has previously received a weak opioid, the initial dose of morphine should be approximately 2 mg/kg/24 hours. If the child has not previously taken weak opioids, the starting dose of morphine sould be reduced accordingly to 1 mg/kg/24 hours.

Doses of strong opioid analgesics

The appropriate doses for the various age groups are set out in Table 9.3.

Table 9.3 Doses of strong opioid analgesics

	Age group				
	0–1	2–5	6–12	13–16	Frequency
Morphine sulphate solution	0.15 mg/kg	3–5 mg	5–10 mg	10–15 mg	4 hrly
Diamorphine hydrochloride	0.1 mg/kg	2–3 mg	3–7 mg	7–10 mg	4 hrly
MST	–	10–15 mg	15–20 mg		
				30 mg	12 hrly

The initial dose should be progressively increased until pain control is achieved titrating morphine dose against pain. Morphine shows no ceiling effect so that an increase in dose will always produce increased analgesia. Bear in mind, however, that failure to control pain despite continually increasing morphine dosage may indicate that the pain is opiate resistant. The nature of the pain should be reassessed and alternative treatment considered.

Typically morphine solution is prescribed initially and the dose increased until a stable dosage is obtained. The dose should be reviewed frequently. This might be twice a day or even at each 4 hourly dose where severe pain requires rapid control. Dose increments of 30–50% are typical:

e.g. morphine 2 mg → 3 mg → 4 mg → 6 mg   4 hourly.

Once pain control is achieved, the dose of morphine solution may be converted to MST if a twice a day schedule is desired. MST and morphine solution appear to be equianalgesic so that the total daily dose of MST will be equal to the total daily dose of morphine solution. Thus a child requiring morphine solution 10 mg 4 hourly (i.e. 60 mg/24 hours) will require MST 30 mg b.d. When changing from morphine solution to MST the last dose of morphine solution and first dose of MST should be given at the same time because of the slow onset of action of MST.

Alternatively, MST may be prescribed from the outset, though morphine solution should also be available for breakthrough pain. The dose of MST is adjusted on a daily basis (or if necessary at each dose). Again increments of 30–50% are usually required. The requirement for breakthrough analgesics over the preceeding 24 hours may give further guidance to the new analgesic requirement. Thus if a child receiving 20 mg of MST b.d. requires four additional doses of morphine solution 5 mg to obtain analgesia, i.e. 60 mg of morphine in total, the next dose of MST should be increased to 30 mg b.d.

Alternative routes of administration

If oral administration of morphine becomes impossible an appropriate alternative route will need to be considered. Morphine suppositories may be useful though they have to be administered every 4 hours. Standard strengths contain 10,15,30 or 60 mg of morphine sulphate or hydrochloride, though the pharmacist can prepare any strength up to 150 mg on request. MST has been used rectally in adults. We have no experience of its use in children and, although it offers the attraction of infrequent administration, absorption may be unreliable.

Morphine and diamorphine have been used by the sublingual or buccal route in adults. This route is of little use in children.

Because of the limitations of the above methods of administration it is preferable to change from oral morphine to s.c. diamorphine by injection or by continuous infusion if repeated injections are anticipated. The dose of oral morphine should be divided by three to give the dose of diamorphine injection. Diamorphine injection is available in 5, 10, 30, 100 and 500 mg ampoules.

Other strong opioids

A variety of other strong opioids are available, e.g. buprenorphine, oxycodone, phenazocine. It is difficult to see that any offers substantial benefits compared to morphine or diamorphine.

Side-effects of opioids

Sedation

This is often feared by parents who feel their child will be 'drugged'.

In fact if appropriate doses are prescribed it occurs in only 20–30% of cases. Moreover any initial sedation usually resolves within 4–5 days. Reassurance on this point is therefore important.

Respiratory depression

Although a theoretical problem, significant respiratory depression is not seen. Should it occur it can be reversed by administration of naloxone (10 mg/kg i.v. or s.c.) though this would seldom seem appropriate.

Constipation

This almost invariably occurs and, unlike other side-effects, tolerance does not develop. Thus prophylactic laxatives should be given to all children on strong opioids.

Nausea and vomiting

This occurs in 25–30% of cases initially. Tolerance develops in 5–10 days in most cases. Haloperidol or cyclizine are helpful if vomiting occurs. Prophylactic prescription of anti-emetics is probably unnecessary.

Hallucinations/confusion

This occurs rarely but is distressing. Tolerance does not develop.

Other side-effects may include difficulty with micturition, dry mouth, sweating and facial flushing. Itching seems to be commoner in children and nasal irritation has been noted in infants.

CO-ANALGESICS

These drugs have little or no intrinsic analgesic activity but none the less produce useful pain relief either alone or as an adjunct to standard analgesic drugs.

Non-steroidal anti-inflammatories (NSAIDs)

These drugs are useful in bone pain and pain due to soft tissue infiltration. Their principal analgesic effect is due to inhibition of the synthesis of prostaglandins. Prostaglandins stimulate osteolysis and mediate bone pain. They also sensitize peripheral nerves. There are many drugs in this class.

Ibuprofen is a relatively weak prostaglandin inhibitor. It has a good side-effect profile, however, and may be used in children over 1 year old. It is available as a suspension (100 mg/5 ml) and as tablets (200 mg, 400 mg and 600 mg). Slow release tablets (800 mg) given daily are also available.

Naproxen and indomethacin are more potent prostaglandin inhibitors and are thus more effective but carry a higher incidence of side-effects, primarily gastric irritation. Naproxen is available as tablets (250 mg and 500 mg), granules (500 mg/sachet), suspension (125 mg/5 ml) and suppositories (500 mg). Indomethacin is available as capsules (25 or 50 mg), modified release tablets (75 mg given once daily), syrup (25 mg/5 ml) and suppositories (100 mg). Diclofenac is available as paediatric suppositories (12.5 mg) but otherwise has no advantage over other anti-inflammatories. It is also available as tablets (25 mg and 50 mg), dispersable tablets (50 mg) and modified release tablets (100 mg) given once daily.

Doses of non-steroidal anti-inflammatories

The appropriate doses for the various age groups are given in Table 9.4.

Table 9.4 Doses of non-steroidal anti-inflammatories

	Age group				Frequency
	0-1	2-5	6-12	13-16	
Ibuprofen	–		20 mg/kg/24 hr		8 hrly
(Junifen					
suspension	–	2.5-5 ml	5-10 ml	10-20 ml	t.i.d.)
Naproxen	–		10 mg/kg/24 hr		12 hrly
Indomethacin	–	–	25 mg b.d.	25 mg t.i.d.	
Diclofenac	–		1-33 mg/kg/24 hr		8 hrly

With more potent NSAIDs it is probably wise to administer an H_2 blocker concurrently because of the risk of gastric irritation. Cimetidine is suitable in doses of 20 mg/kg/24 hours (suspension 200 mg/5 ml or tablets 200 and 400 mg).

Corticosteroids

Steroids have a number of applications in terminal illness. Their use in anorexia is considered elsewhere (p. 147). They are also useful as co-analgesics, for example in headache due to raised ICP, or pain due to bone invasion or nerve compression. The dose used in these circumstances is higher than that used for anorexia. Bear in mind when considering steroids that steroid-induced Cushingoid features may be particularly severe in children and are often distressing to the family. If steroids are prescribed and little benefit is obtained they should be stopped, particularly if alternative treatment is available. Where benefits of treatment are substantial the dose should be reduced to the minimum required to control symptoms at the earliest opportunity.

Dexamethasone is usually used and is available as tablets (500 μg and 2 mg) and injection (4 mg/ml). A suspension (4 mg/5 ml) may be prepared by the pharmacist. The dosage is as shown in Table 9.5.

Table 9.5 Doses of dexamethasone

	Age group				
	0–1	2–5	6–12	13–16	Frequency
High dose – (e.g. ICP, bone pain, nerve compression)	–	2 mg	3 mg	4–16 mg	12 hrly
Low dose – (anorexia)	–	0.5–1 mg	1–2 mg	2–4 mg	Once daily

Prednisolone is an alternative to dexamethasone and prednisolone soluble tablets (Prednesol 5 mg) may be useful. Prednisolone 7 mg is equivalent to 1 mg of dexamethasone.

The last dose of steroid should be given 5–6 hours before bed time if possible to avoid insomnia. Like non-steroidal anti-inflammatories steroids may produce gastric irritation but H_2 blockers are generally unnecessary.

Antidepressants

These may be helpful for deafferentation pain where the pain has a burning quality. Imipramine is suitable. Dosage and presentation are as for depression (see p. 157).

Anticonvulsants

These may be helpful where deafferentation pain is of stabbing quality. Carbamazepine or sodium valproate are used.

Carbamazepine is available as tablets (100 mg, 200 mg and 400 mg) and as an elixir (100 mg/5 ml).

Sodium valproate is available as crushable tablets (100 mg), enteric coated tablets (200 mg and 500 mg) and elixir (200 mg/5 ml).

For dosages according to age group see Table 9.6.

Table 9.6 Doses of anticonvulsants

	Age group				
	0–1	2–5	6–12	13–16	Frequency
Carbamaze-pine	100–200 mg/ 24 hr	200–400 mg/ 24 hr	400–600 mg/ 24 hr	600–1000 mg/ 24 hr	b.d. or t.i.d.
Sodium valproate		Initially 10 mg/kg/24 hr Increased to 20–30 mg/ kg/24 hr			b.d.

Muscle relaxants

Baclofen, diazepam or dantrolene may relieve pain caused by skeletal muscle spasm. Their use is discussed further elsewhere (p. 158).

Anxiolytics

Fear and anxiety often play an important part in 'total pain'. When reassurance or distraction prove insufficient anxiolytic drugs may help. Haloperidol, diazepam and chlorpromazine are suitable and are discussed further below (pp. 155–6).

OTHER ANALGESIC TECHNIQUES

Radiotherapy

Palliative radiotherapy is the treatment of choice for isolated bone secondaries. A single treatment is often effective within 7–10 days. Widespread bone metastases present more of a problem.

Nerve blocks

These specialized techniques may produce good relief of pain where other techniques have failed, such as pain due to nerve destruction/ invasion. They are used infrequently in paediatric terminal care. This in part reflects the different pathology seen in children, where solid tumour invasion of nerve trunks is less common than in adults. It also perhaps reflects the difficulty in arriving at a precise neuro-anatomical diagnosis in children and technical problems such as achieving sufficient cooperation to perform the block.

CNS opiates

Opiates may be administered directly into the CNS via an epidural catheter, either by intermittent injection or continuous infusion. This has the advantage of limiting the opiate dosage and therefore reducing side-effects. This is most likely to be of value in situations where intractable pain requires large, constantly increasing doses of opiates leading to continuing sedation, as for example in osteosarcoma with multiple bone metastases.

Transcutaneous nerve stimulation (TNS)

TNS is thought to work by stimulating endogeous opiate release at spinal level or by 'closing the pain gate' effectively inhibiting transmission of pain. It may be useful in older children with mild pain but is of limited value.

NAUSEA AND VOMITING

Nausea and vomiting are common and often coexist, often sharing a common cause. Although vomiting is the more dramatic, nausea is often more distressing. Vomiting once or twice per day is often acceptable, persisting nausea is not. There are many possible causes of nausea and vomiting and the likely mechanism should be considered before initiating treatment. This stage is easily overlooked and as a consequence one anti-emetic after another is prescribed, singly or in combination, until control is achieved more by accident than design.

Mechanism of vomiting

Figure 9.2 summarizes the principal pathways leading to vomiting.

Causes of vomiting

The cause of vomiting can often be deduced from a knowledge of the disease process involved, enquiry about the nature of vomiting and the circumstances in which it occurs, and the presence of associated symptoms such as headache or constipation. The drug history may provide further clues, cytotoxics or opiates may, for example, be responsible. Examination may reveal signs such as papilloedema or a loaded colon.

In children the more common causes of vomiting include:

(a) constipation;
(b) raised intracranial pressure;
(c) excessive pharyngeal secretions (see p. 153).

While constipation is common, obstruction is rare, reflecting the rarity of gastrointestinal tumours. One unusual situation in which obstruction may occur is in lymphoma where enlarged lymphatic tissue in the bowel wall may act as the focus for an intussusception.

Vomiting due to raised intracranial pressure often presents a characteristic picture of effortless, projectile vomiting. Having vomited,

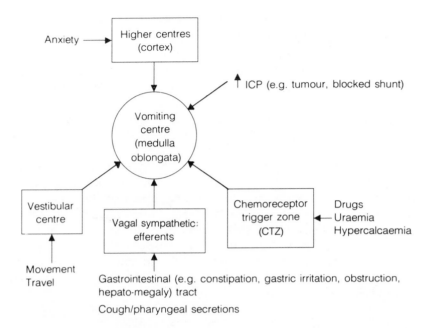

Fig 9.2 Causes of vomiting.

the child is often free of the nausea that lingers in other forms of vomiting. It can be successfully treated with high dose steroids, though if it is infrequent and does not interfere with other treatment or distress the child unduly, the 'knee-jerk' response of steroids for raised pressure should be resisted. Steroid side-effects will probably be severe.

Available drugs

Drugs should be selected according to the cause of vomiting and should have an appropriate site of action (see above). Where possible, a single drug should be used. If combinations of anti-emetics are required they should be chosen from groups acting at different sites.

Oral treatment is preferred but not always possible. In general if the frequency of vomiting is three or more times per day an alternative route of administration should be chosen. This is influenced by other factors such as the degree of distress caused by vomiting and the effect of vomiting on the administration of other treatment. Repeated i.m. injections should be avoided. Treatment by suppository, s.c. injection or s.c. infusion is preferred. Often other drug treatment can be continued by mouth. Rectal or parenteral anti-emetics may be converted to oral equivalents when control is achieved.

It is helpful to classify the principal drugs used according to their main site of action.

Drugs acting on the chemo-receptor trigger zone

Haloperidol is perhaps the most helpful drug in this class. It has additional anxiolytic activity and the incidence of extra-pyramidal side-effects is low. It is available as tablets (500 µg and 1.5 mg), liquid (1 mg/ml and 2 mg/ml) and injection (5 mg/ml). The injection is suitable for s.c. or i.m. use.

Chlorpromazine is more sedating and is too irritant to use by s.c. injection. Crushing the tablets should be avoided because of the risk of contact sensitivity. It is available as tablets (10 mg, 25 mg, 50 mg and 100 mg), syrup (25 mg/5 ml), injection (25 mg/ml) and suppositories (100 mg as standard or 12.5/25 mg by special request). If suppositories are used 100 mg is equivalent to 40–50 mg given orally.

Prochlorperazine is less sedating than chlorpromazine but tends to produce extra-pyramidal side-effects in children. Again it is too irritant to be used by s.c. injection. The suppository may be useful. It is available as tablets (5 mg), syrup (5 mg/5 ml), injection (12.5 mg/ml) and suppositories (5 mg and 25 mg). If the suppositories are used, 5 mg is roughly equivalent to 2.5 mg given orally.

Drugs acting on the vomiting centre

Cyclizine is the principal drug in this class. It may be sedating in high doses but is usually well tolerated. It is suitable for s.c. administration. It is available as tablets (50 mg), injection (50 mg/ml) and suppositories (50 mg) on a named patient basis.

Drugs acting on the gastrointestinal tract

Domperidone is the most useful drug in this class, lacking the troublesome central side-effects of metoclopramide. It is available as tablets (10 mg), suspension (5 mg/5 ml) and suppositories (30 mg or lower strengths by arrangement with the pharmacist). If the suppository is used, 30 mg is equivalent to 10 mg given orally.*

Metoclopramide has a reputation for producing extra-pyramidal side-effects in children and adolescents and is generally best avoided. It may none the less prove useful on occasions. The injection may be given s.c.

Dosage of anti-emetics

Dosages of the various anti-emetics are set out in Table 9.7.

ANOREXIA

This is commonly reported in malignant disease. The cause is often obscure. It may be associated with nausea and vomiting, in which

---

* Current UK Licence for Domperidone limits its use in children to Chemo/Radiotherapy-Induced Vomiting.

Table 9.7 Dosage of anti-emetics

| | \multicolumn{4}{c}{Age group} | |
	0–1	2–5	6–12	13–16	Frequency
Haloperidol	25 µg/kg	200 µg	400 µg	1.5 mg	b.i.d.
Chlor-promazine	–	500 µg/kg	10 mg	25–50 mg	t.i.d.
Prochlor-perazine	–	1.25–2.5 mg	2.5–5 mg	5–10 mg	t.i.d.
Cyclizine	1 mg/kg	12.5 mg	25 mg	50 mg	t.i.d.
Domperidone	0.1 mg/kg	1 mg	5 mg	10 mg	t.i.d.
Metoclo-pramide	1 mg b.d.	1–2 mg t.i.d.	2.5–5 mg t.i.d.	5–10 mg t.i.d.	

case appropriate anti-emetic treatment may relieve it. It may also be associated with pain, anxiety or depression.

Anorexia tends to distress parents more than children. Parents are often anxious, even in the late stages of illness, that they are failing to supply their child's nutritional needs. Reassurance may be helpful. It is worth explaining that energy requirements are reduced with inactivity – that their child does not need much food because he is doing very little. Enquiry about favourite foods and specific dislikes will suggest which meals will be most palatable. Remember that the sense of taste is often altered, so that meat, for example, often tastes bitter. Do not assume that sweet foods will necessarily appeal to children. Offering small frequent snacks is more likely to meet with success than a plate full of food and an invitation to 'eat what you can and leave the rest'.

The only therapeutic measure available to alleviate anorexia is prescription of a small dose of steroids. This is seldom warranted because of the problems of steroid side-effects and the dubious benefits of treatment, particularly where anorexia does not bother the child. Appropriate dosage is described in the section on co-analgesics.

CONSTIPATION

Constipation is a common symptom in both malignant and non-malignant terminal illness. It is often overlooked or underestimated by parents and carers alike. Children may not readily admit to constipation because of embarrassment or fear of the consequences – previous complaint may have led to an enema. Bed or chair-bound children may find constipation convenient as it avoids the need for transfer to the toilet, which may be difficult or painful. In the incontinent child constipation may temporarily maintain continence until, of course, overflow supervenes. Overflow is commonly misinterpreted as true faecal incontinence so that treatment with anti-diarrhoeals worsens the situation.

The cause of constipation is often complex. Typically it is precipitated by immobility aided and abetted by reduced food and fluid intake.

Drugs, particularly opiate analgesics, often compound the problem. The constipated child, if communicative, may reveal the problem directly. Other presentations include abdominal pain, nausea, vomiting, anorexia or agitation.

Constipation is so common it should be actively sought in all dying children. Treatment should be initiated early and should be oral whenever possible. The starting dose of oral treatment may be increased until constipation is controlled or side-effects, such as griping with contact laxatives, limit further increment. If combinations of laxatives are used it is logical to use drugs from different therapeutic groups, such as a contact laxative and a faecal softener. By commencing adequate oral treatment at the appropriate time impaction and consequent need for rectal treatments may be avoided. This is particularly true in circumstances where constipation is predictable. It is worth reiterating the need for prophylactic laxatives with opiates, where constipation follows as surely as night follows day.

Oral laxatives

These may be broadly divided into two groups, contact, or stimulant, laxatives and osmotic, or softening, laxatives. Some drugs combine both properties.

Contact laxatives

Danthron is available in two main forms. Codanthramer suspension is useful in children and is available as standard (25 mg danthron in 5 ml) and forte (75 mg danthron in 5 ml) suspensions. The initial dose is 12.5 – 25 mg daily. Codanthrusate capsules are useful in older children and combine danthron (50 mg) with docusate (60 mg). The initial dose is one to two capsules daily. The onset of action is typically 8–12 hours after administration.

Bisacodyl is available as 5 mg tablets and also as paediatric (5 mg) and standard (10 mg) suppositories. The usual dose of tablets is 5 mg daily. It usually acts in approximately 12 hours.

Docusate has combined stimulant and softening properties. It has a somewhat slower onset of action however (24–48 hours). It is available as a solution (12.5 or 50 mg/5 ml). Usual dose in children older than 6 months is 12.5–25 mg t.i.d.

Senna acts in 8–12 hours. It is available as tablets, granules and syrup. Children between 2 and 6 years old are best treated with syrup 2.5–5 ml daily. Children between 6 and 12 years may be given 5–10 ml of syrup, one to two tablets or a 5 ml level spoonful of granules, mixed with a drink, daily. Children over 12 years will require 10–20 ml of syrup, two to four tablets or two 5 ml level spoonfuls of granules daily.

(Note: 10 ml senna syrup = 10 ml codanthramer forte syrup
                      = 3 codanthrusate capsules.)

Osmotic laxatives

Lactulose is the principal agent in this group. Its onset of action is slower than that of the contact laxatives (36–48 hours). Many children find its taste sickly. It is available as a solution and is given twice daily in initial doses of: 0–1 year 2.5 ml; 2–5 years 5 ml; 6–12 years 10 ml; and over 12 years 15 ml.

Rectal treatment

If the child presents with impaction or becomes impacted despite oral treatment then rectal measures will be required to clear the lower bowel. This should, of course, be followed by initiation of oral laxatives if none were previously prescribed or alteration of the pre-existing laxative regime. The guide to lower bowel clearance in impaction is rectal examination. The simple flow chart in Figure 9.3 covers most instances.

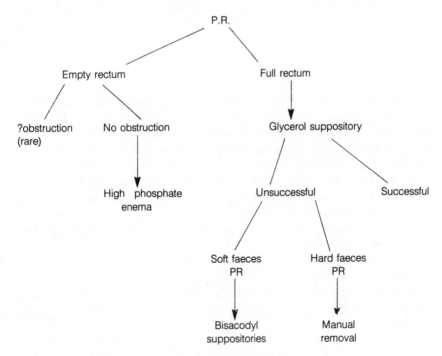

Fig. 9.3 Treatment of impaction of the lower bowel.

Note:
(a) Glycerol suppositories are suitable for children of all ages, being available in infant, child and standard adult sizes.
(b) Docusate enema is an alternative to phosphate enema for children over 3 years of age. Sodium citrate (Micralax) is another option.
(c) A manual removal is distressing and should only be performed after application of topical anaesthetic gel and, if necessary, administration of sedation.

DYSPNOEA

Mechanism of dyspnoea

Respiration is controlled by the brain stem respiratory centre under neuronal/chemical control. Factors such as lowered blood O_2 tension, raised CO_2 tension or increased H^+ concentration are the principal physical factors which lead to an increased respiratory drive and hence the feeling of shortness of breath. This is, however, simplistic and dyspnoea is in fact a more complex subjective experience influenced by the presence or absence of factors such as fear, anxiety and pain.

Causes of dyspnoea

In children a wide variety of disease processes may lead to dyspnoea. Cardiopulmonary disease is less common than in adults. Congenital heart disease and cystic fibrosis are perhaps the commonest examples. Primary lung tumours are rare but secondaries from tumours such as osteosarcoma or Wilm's tumour may occur. Effusions may be seen with lymphoma and other malignancies. Respiratory muscle dysfunction in children with neurodegenerative disease such as spinal muscular atrophy or muscular dystrophy is relatively common. A chest infection complicating the primary illness is often to blame.

Dyspnoea due to cerebral tumours, with raised intracranial pressure or direct respiratory centre invasion, may also be seen.

Anaemia in relapsed leukaemia or uraemia in renal failure secondary to problems such as cystinosis, or polycystic kidneys, may also be responsible.

Treatment

Treatment may be aimed at the underlying cause, if treatment is likely to improve symptomatology, or at the dyspnoea itself.

Treatment of the cause

Heart failure may be treated with diuretics with useful palliation of symptoms. Often, however, general measures (see below) are equally helpful.

Treatment of chest infections in the late stage of an illness raises difficult questions. Antibiotics may lessen symptoms and therefore be regarded as a reasonable palliative measure. However, more rapid palliation can often be achieved by other therapies which should not be withheld while benefit from antibiotics is awaited. Ultimately the decision is determined by the wishes of the parents, who may feel that failure to treat with antibiotics may shorten their child's life. No matter how long their child's illness, no matter how many times they have discussed what they might do in these circumstances, when the time comes the decision is agonizing. It is difficult to know how far to guide parents – ultimately the decision must be one that they feel comfortable with not forced into. At the same time one often senses that they might welcome a direct and unequivocal instruction to relieve them of the burden. Certainly it is worth stressing that, at such a late stage in the illness, antibiotics are unlikely to influence life expectancy significantly. It is also worth telling the parents, who will often express a dread of making the 'wrong' decision, that there is no right or wrong decision to make. The decision is rather the one with which they feel most comfortable. If the parents do chose antibiotic therapy, most will accept that only oral treatment is appropriate so that, as and when the child becomes unable to take treatment by mouth, antibiotics may be abandoned.

Anaemia, most commonly seen in relapsed leukaemia, may be treated by transfusion. Particularly where the disease is progressing rapidly transfusion is best avoided. Transfusion is painful, inhibits contact, and because of changes occurring in stored blood does not give immediate benefit. Moreover, profound anaemia, with its progressive tiredness and eventual coma, may be corrected only for the child to die from a distressing terminal haemorrhage.

Significant pleural effusions are rarely seen, for example in lymphoma. If present, consideration should be given to a pleural tap.

Empirical treatment of dyspnoea

Often dyspnoea and anxiety co-exist – one symptom fuelling the other. Thus relief of anxiety by providing a reassuring atmosphere, with parents or a trusted care team member present, and, if necessary, anxiolytic drugs, is helpful.

Opiates reduce anxiety and alleviate pain, which itself can lead to dyspnoea. In addition, opiates have a specific effect on the respiratory centre, reducing its sensitivity to changes in blood O_2 and CO_2 tensions. They can, therefore, produce significant improvement in dyspnoea regardless of its cause. Usually smaller doses are required than those given for analgesic effect. Typically about half the dose will be required. Morphine elixir, or diamorphine injection, should be used rather than MST.

Oxygen may give some relief over the short term but is not terribly helpful. Children find oxygen giving sets frightening and the presence of tubing, mask and cylinder prevent physical contact.

Anxiolytics may alleviate dyspnoea by reducing associated anxiety and possibly by reducing respiratory muscle tone, so relieving the feeling of 'tightness'. They may potentially cause respiratory depression, as may opiates, but this is not usually of practical significance in the terminal phase of an illness. Oral diazepam is suitable, but rectal diazepam solution is more rapid in onset for acute dyspnoea.

Nebulized bronchodilators (e.g. salbutamol 2.5–5 mg 4–6 hourly) occasionally prove helpful. Corticosteroids are rarely of value, bronchial obstruction and lymphangitis being uncommon in children.

COUGH

This is perhaps more common than one might imagine and may be accompanied by dyspnoea as they share a number of common causes, such as cystic fibrosis, heart failure or secondary lung deposits. Cough due to retained secretions is extremely common in children with neurodegenerative disorders. Pharyngeal muscle involvement leads to pooling of secretions in the upper airways, while respiratory muscle involvement produces an ineffectual cough. Aspiration of medication or feeds is common in these circumstances. Respiratory infections complicating the primary illness may also be responsible for coughs.

Treatment may be directed at the underlying cause, for example prescribing antibiotics for respiratory infection or hyoscine to dry excessive secretions. Gentle physiotherapy and suction may be of value. Vigorous physiotherapy is inappropriate and may be distressing. Humidified air may ease a dry cough but the administration equipment may frighten the child.

If the cough is painful or distressing, and particularly if it disturbs sleep, cough suppressant drugs may help. Cough suppressants may work by:

1. Peripheral suppression. Simple linctus is a soothing preparation available as paediatric simple linctus for use in younger children. Doses of 5–10 ml may be repeated as frequently as required.

2. Central suppression. Opiates produce central suppression of the cough reflex. Codeine linctus is appropriate in initial doses of approximately half those used for analgaesia (see Table 9.2). The initial dose may be increased to the full therapeutic dose if necessary. Morphine, or diamorphine, linctus may be used if codeine is unsuccessful. Again, starting doses of approximately half those used for analgaesia (see Table 9.3) are appropriate. The dose may be increased until control is achieved.

Massive haemoptysis is thankfully a rare event but, like massive haematemesis, may sometimes occur in the presence of a bleeding diathesis, as in relapsed leukaemia. Catastrophic terminal bleeding is terrifying for the child to experience and horrendous for the family to witness. The only available treatment is rapid sedation. It is perhaps one of the few situations where intravenous therapy is warranted and if venous access is already established or readily obtainable i.v diamorphine and diazepam, repeated if necessary, will help. Alternatively rectal diazepam and s.c. diamorphine may be given if venous access is not immediately available. Provision of red towels and blankets may reduce distress by concealing the extent of blood loss.

NOISY BREATHING

Retained secretions

These may be present in children with neurodegenerative disease from a relatively early stage, as described above. In other diseases they become a problem only in the last hours of life and present the familiar 'death rattle'. This is often distressing to parents and warrants treatment. Hyoscine is usually effective and in the terminal situation is administered as an s.c injection at a dose of 15µg/kg. It may be repeated 4 hourly or administered via an s.c. infusion pump. Hyoscine's sedative effect will generally be a welcome additional benefit – though repeated doses may produce a paradoxical agitation.

The use of hyoscine over longer periods in children with neurodegenerative disease is more contentious. It may be administered orally in the form of hyoscine tablets (300 and 600µg or by sustained release hyoscine patches (Scopaderm TTS) which release some 500µg of hyoscine over 72 hours. The usual dose of oral hyoscine is: 4–10 years 75–150µg 6 hourly, over 10 years 150–300µg 6 hourly. The relatively low but constant dosage supplied by the TTS system seems equally effective, one patch is generally sufficient in the under 10s while two patches may be required simultaneously in older children. The patch is usually effective for 48–72 hours. Potential problems with repeated use of hyoscine include sedation, urinary retention, constipation and paralytic ileus. Our experience has been that these do not occur when hyoscine patches are used – though caution is still required.

Grunting respiration

Grunting laboured respiration may occur in the late stages of illness – usually in a deeply unconscious child. It often distresses parents and may be eased by administration of rectal diazepam 5–10 mg. If dyspnoea is also present, diamorphine in appropriate dosage by s.c. injection may be of benefit.

FITS

Fits are commonly encountered in terminal childhood illness, reflecting the prevalance of conditions such as primary cerebral tumours and CNS degenerative disease. A detailed account of long-term treatment of fits is beyond the scope of this chapter. It is worth commenting, however, that in the presence of structural or metabolic abnormality of the brain, fit control is likely to be poor and multiple drug regimes the norm. Often progression of the disease, particularly in the later stages, is accompanied by deterioration in fit control.

Parents have often, therefore, had a great deal of experience of fits and usually accept them with a considerable degree of calm. Minor or short-lived fits generally require no specific treatment. If prolonged, major seizures occur, administration of rectal diazepam is the usual first line of treatment. Rectal solution should be used rather than suppositories which are too slowly absorbed. Rectal solution is available as 5 or 10 mg/2.5 ml. If rectal solution is unavailable, diazepam injection may be drawn up and administered rectally via a quill. Diazepam may also be given by i.v. injection, though venous access may prove difficult in a fitting child. It should not be used i.m. as the onset of action is too slow. Diazepam injection is available in 10 mg/2 ml ampoules.

If initial diazepam fails to control the fit it may be repeated after 5–10 minutes. If diazepam is still unsuccessful paraldehyde should be tried. It is usually successful and provides a longer duration of fit control, and sedation, than diazepam. Although it may be given i.m., rectal administration is preferred. A glass syringe should be used and the paraldehyde diluted with an equal volume of arachis oil before administration via a quill. The dose may be repeated if necessary. (For dosages see Table 9.8.)

Table 9.8 Dosage of drugs used for emergency control of fits

	Age group			
	1	1-5	6-12	13-16
Diazepam	2.5 mg	5 mg	5-10 mg	10 mg
Paraldehyde	0.1 ml/kg	1 ml per year of age	5 ml + 0.5 ml for each year	10 ml

PSYCHOLOGICAL SYMPTOMS

This loose term encompasses anxiety, agitation, depression and insomnia. Although each will be considered separately, they often co-exist so the distinction is somewhat artificial.

Anxiety

Anxiety is most commonly encountered at the time of diagnosis, at times of crisis, such as relapse of disease, and when it becomes clear that cure is not possible and death is inevitable. During the course of the terminal stage of the illness anxiety is likely to be most marked at the time of appearance of new and unfamiliar symptoms. It is experienced by both the child and the family, particularly the parents. Each will have their own fears and concerns.

Provision of time to discuss their anxieties is of prime importance. Sometimes fears will be groundless and reassurance can be total. More often there is a rational basis for their fear and it will not be possible to allay it completely. A degree of reassurance is none the less possible in most cases. Thus, for example, we may not be able to say that pain will not occur but will be able to say, that if it does occur we will be able to respond to it and usually control it. Diversion is also important. Fear tends to expand to fill the time made available to it. Purposeful occupation of otherwise empty hours is thus essential. Even dying children need to play.

Where discussion and diversion are insufficient, the use of anxiolytic drugs should be considered, but their prescription should be an adjunct to, rather than a substitute for, listening and appropriate reassurance. Sometimes their prescription will allow a child to discuss a subject previously too frightening to talk about. It is best to start with small doses of anxiolytics to avoid initial side-effects such as excessive sedation, which may make the drug unacceptable to the child or his parents.

Haloperidol is useful as it is relatively non-sedating and extra-pyramidal side-effects are usually only a problem at higher doses. Its anti-emetic action may be useful. It is available as a liquid (1 mg and 2 mg/ml), tablets (500μg and 1.5 mg) and s.c. or i.m. injection (5 mg/ml).

Chlorpromazine is more sedating. Again extra-pyramidal side-effects may be seen at high doses. It shares haloperidol's anti-emetic activity. It is available as a syrup (25 mg/5 ml), tablets (10 mg, 25 mg, 50 mg and 100 mg), i.m. injection (25 mg/ml) and suppositories (12.5, 25 and 100 mg).

Diazepam is also sedating. Its long half-life means that a single daily dose is often adequate, but it tends to accumulate. Paradoxical agitation occurs in some children so that if anxiety seems to be increasing, despite diazepam, an alternative drug should be employed. Diazepam is available as an elixir (2 mg/5 ml), tablets (2 mg, 5 mg and 10 mg), rectal solution (5 and 10 mg) suppositories (10 mg) and i.m. or i.v. injection (5 mg/ml).

Starting doses are indicated in Table 9.9.

Table 9.9 Starting doses of anxiolytics

	Age group				Frequency
	0–1	2–5	6–12	13–16	
Haloperidol	25 μg/kg	200 μg	400 μg	1.5 mg	b.d.
Chlorpromazine	–	500 μg/kg	10–25 mg	25–50 mg	t.i.d.
Diazepam	200 μg/kg	2–4 mg	5–10 mg	10–40 mg	o.d. (nocte)

Agitation

The agitated child is frightened and restless and requires speedy assessment and treatment. Sometimes an underlying cause, such as constipation, urinary retention or pain, may be identified and should be treated appropriately. If no cause is found, empirical treatment with anxiolytics should be instituted as soon as possible.

The oral doses of anxiolytics described above may be repeated hourly until the child settles. Sedation is usually acceptable in these circumstances so that diazepam or chlorpromazine are useful.

If the child is unable to take oral medication, diazepam administered as rectal solution is rapidly acting and usually effective. Chlorpromazine is too irritant to give subcutaneously and intramuscular injection is painful. Haloperidol given s.c. is an alternative.

Methotrimeprazine (Nozinan) is also effective by s.c. injection in doses of 12.5–25 mg every 6 hours in children over 12 years.

Insomnia

There are many possible causes of insomnia. The child's sleep pattern may have been disturbed by frequent hospital admissions. He may be in pain. He may simply be too frightened to sleep in case he fails to wake. Often the problem is complex. Whatever the cause, insomnia is disruptive and destroys the morale of the child and family. If a specific cause can be identified, it should be remedied. If no cause is apparent and insomnia persists it may be helped by prescription of an appropriate hypnotic.

Diazepam may be used but its prolonged action and subsequent day time sedation limit its usefulness. Temazepam has a shorter half-life and is more useful. It is available as an oral solution (10 mg/5 ml), tablets (10 mg and 20 mg) and capsules (10, 15, 20 and 30 mg).

Chloral hydrate and its derivative triclofos are useful hypnotics in younger children. Triclofos is preferable as it causes less gastric irritation than chloral. Chloral is available as chloral mixture (500 mg/5ml) and chloral paediatric mixture (200 mg/5 ml). Both should be taken well diluted with water or milk. Tablets (414 mg chloral hydrate) and capsules (500 mg) are also available but are not recommended for use in children. Triclofos elixir contains 500 mg triclofos/5 ml.

Promethazine is a sedating antihistamine preparation. It is available as tablets (10 mg and 25 mg) and an elixir (5 mg/ml). For dosages of all these drugs, see Table 9.10.

Table 9.10 Doses of hypnotics*

	Age group			
	0–1	1–5	6–12	13–16
Temazepam	400 µg/kg	4–8 mg	10–20 mg	20–40 mg
Chloral	200 mg	250–500 mg	500–1000 mg	1000–2000 mg
Triclofos	100–250 mg	250–500 mg	500–1000 mg	1000–2000 mg
Promethazine	5–10 mg	10–20 mg	20–25 mg	25–50 mg

* Once daily at bedtime.

Depression

Sadness is, understandably, common in children with terminal illness; true depression is rare. It is seen more often in the child's family than in the child. When it does occur it may go unrecognized for a number of reasons. Children may fail to express their emotions in a way that adults might recognize as depression. Other clues to its presence, such as sleep disturbance, loss of appetite and loss of interest in normal activities, may readily be attributed to the terminal illness itself.

The diagnosis of depression is therefore often difficult and expert advice may be required. If it is recognized and treatment instituted it is likely to be 10–14 days before benefit is seen, though some features, such as sleep disturbance, may improve more quickly.

A tricyclic antidepressant such as imipramine is usually prescribed. It is available as a syrup (25 mg/5 ml) and as tablets (10 mg and 25 mg) and is suitable for use in children in the following doses:

0–4 yr	5–12 yr	13–16 yr	Frequency
–	10 mg	25 mg	t.i.d.

MUSCLE SPASM

Muscle spasm is a significant cause of pain in paediatric terminal illness. Its treatment is outlined on p. 132. Note that the relief of spasm may produce problems of its own. Motor function may depend on a degree of spasticity so that its relief may render the child less able to assist with transfer etc. Relief of the pain, which is unresponsive to analgesics, is, none the less, of prime importance, even if it is achieved by the sacrifice of some residual locomotor ability.

Available drugs

Baclofen is often effective, though sedation may be troublesome with higher doses. Occasionally a paradoxical increase in spasm is seen. It is available as syrup (5 mg/5 ml) and tablets (10 mg). A small initial dose of 0.75–2 mg/kg/24 hours is increased every 2 days until control is achieved. Usual maximum daily doses are: 1–5 years 30 mg/day, 6–8 years 40 mg/day, 9–12 years 60 mg/day, 13–16 years 100 mg/day. Doses are given on a t.i.d basis.

Diazepam may also be useful. It acts quickly but again produces sedation. Small starting doses should therefore be used. Doses and preparations are outlined in the section on control of anxiety (p. 156).

Dantrolene is of limited value. Benefits of treatment are often not seen for several weeks. It should be avoided in younger children. In adolescents the usual starting dose is 25 mg increased at weekly intervals to a maximum of 100 mg q.i.d. It is available only as dantrolene capsules (25 mg).

TREATMENT IN THE LAST HOURS/DAYS

The final stage of a terminal illness is characterized by decreased consciousness and increased dependency. The child's requirement for physical care is high as are the emotional stakes for the family. Their experiences in the last moments of their child's life may have a profound effect on their subsequent reaction to bereavement. Skilful management of symptoms is therefore of great importance.

Additional treatment may be required for new symptoms, such as agitation or 'death rattle'. Existing treatment will need to be rationalized as oral treatment becomes more difficult and ultimately alternative routes of administration may need to be considered. Some oral therapy may reasonably be abandoned; some will require the substitution of an equivalent parenteral or rectal drug.

Drugs that may usually be discontinued at this stage include:

Steroids.
NSAIDs.
Laxatives.
Antibiotics.
Mild (non-opioid) analgesics.

Drugs that will require substitution include:

Opioid analgesics: Both weak and strong opioids should be changed to diamorphine by s.c. injection or infusion. Morphine suppositories are an alternative.
Anticonvulsants: Change to rectal diazepam 4–6 hourly. Rectal peraldehyde may be of additional value.
Anti-emetics: Change to haloperidol or cyclizine by s.c. infusion. Metoclopramide may also be used by s.c. infusion but at the risk of extra-pyramidal side-effects. Domperidone, chlorpromazine or prochlorperazine suppositories are alternatives.
Psychotropics: Haloperidol, or methotrimeprazine in older children, are suitable for s.c. infusion. Rectal diazepam or chlorpromazine are alternatives.

SUBCUTANEOUS INFUSION PUMPS

Continuous subcutaneous infusion offers an excellent means of drug administration when oral treatment is no longer possible. A number of infusion pumps are available. All deliver the solution contained in the syringe at a preset rate so that a constant amount of drug is administered over the duration of the infusion. Some have a boost facility which allows small fixed bolus doses to be administered. The Graseby infusion pump (MS26) is perhaps the most popular of this type.

The pump is connected to a 23G s.c. butterfly needle via infusion tubing. The butterfly cannula is inserted subcutaneously, usually on the chest or abdominal wall or the upper arm or thigh. Areas of broken or oedematous skin should be avoided. The needle and a loop of infusion tubing should be secured with 'Opsite' or a similar dressing to avoid accidental removal. The pumps are portable and may be carried in a 'holster' if the child is mobile. They are relatively unobtrusive and do not usually impair contact. The site can usually be maintained for up to a week – and sometimes as much as 2 weeks. Induration is common at the infusion site and should not necessitate a change of site, unless inflammation or discomfort are present.

Drugs suitable for subcutaneous infusion

Analgesics: diamorphine is preferred to morphine because of its greater solubility. Diamorphine remains stable in syringes for up to 3 weeks. **Anti-emetics**: cyclizine and haloperidol are suitable. Both tend to crystalize and precipitate in higher concentrations, particularly if kept in the syringe for long periods of time. Low concentrations should therefore be used (25 mg/ml in the case of cyclizine and 2 mg/ml in the case of haloperidol). Cyclizine is more likely to precipitate if mixed with diamorphine. Haloperidol tends to be degraded by light.

Hyoscine is primarily used to reduce secretions but has additional anti-emetic activity. It appears to be very stable.

Methotrimeprazine produces additional sedation. It may be irritant in higher concentrations.

Metoclopramide is degraded by light, though this is only likely to be of significance in infusions of several days' duration.

Chlorpromazine, prochlorperazine, diazepam and dexamethasone are potent irritants and should **not** be used subcutaneously.

Preparing infusion solutions

The contents of the infusion pump will obviously vary according to symptom control requirements. However, a few general points are worth bearing in mind:

(a) Avoid using more than two drugs. Interactions will be more likely if more drugs are used. Using drugs which serve a dual purpose may help to limit the number of drugs required, such as haloperidol for the anxious, vomiting child.

(b) Keep drug concentrations low. This may help to avoid precipitation, particularly with anti-emetic/analgesic combinations.

(c) Limit the infusion time to 24 hours.

(d) Keep the infusion out of direct light.

(e) Remember to take into account the volume of solution required to prime the infusion tubing when first establishing the infusion. This is usually approximately 1.5 ml. This 'dead volume' will not be delivered by the syringe driver. Thus if it is intended to infuse 10 ml of solution/24 hours and 10 ml of solution is prepared, only 8.5 ml will be available for infusion, once 1.5 ml has been used to prime the tubing. The infusion will therefore be completed in approximately 20 hours, so that the infusion started at 9 am and expected to run until 9 am the next morning will need to be changed at 5 am. Clearly this presents particular problems in the community where nursing or medical staff are not immediately available.

(f) Likewise if an alteration is made in the syringe regime the infusion tubing should be reprimed with the new solution. If it is not, it is likely to be several hours before the child receives the altered treatment.

(g) Setting the infusion rate on the infusion pump can be an important source of error. The infusion rate on the popular Graseby models, for example, is defined in mm/hour and corresponds to the millimetre scale marked on the side of the pump. The rate does not correspond to the millilitre scale on the syringe barrel. For standard 10 ml Gillette or Braun Omnifix syringes, the length of the barrel to 10 ml is 50 mm, so that setting a rate of 50 mm/24 hours (on the Graseby MS26) will deliver 10 ml of solution/24 hours. With other syringes the required volume should be drawn up and measured against the mm scale to give the corresponding infusion rate in mm/24 hours.

Infusion rates on other machines are calculated differently. It is probably best to be familiar with one machine and use it exclusively.

CHAPTER 10

Terminal care at home – the practical issues

Sharon Beardsmore and Sue Alder

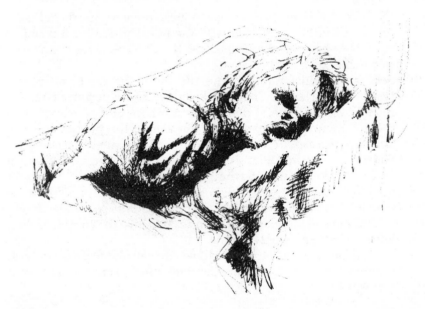

If this book has one major theme it is that no aspect of caring for a dying child and his family can be taken in isolation. Physical care cannot be separated from emotional support and the child cannot be cared for without his family's needs being addressed. Without losing sight of this holistic approach, contributors have focused on specific areas where specialist skills and knowledge can be applied to assist the family. This chapter highlights the particular problems faced by families caring for their child at home, and identifies practical ways in which professionals can contribute towards an ultimately peaceful death for the child and support for the family.

Once the decision of where to care for the child has been taken there are a number of continuing issues to be considered. These include the type of support required, communication with and between professionals; respite from caring; concerns about physical symptoms and the mode of death; supply of equipment and medicines; and the question of continuing treatment.

The authors have particular expertise with children suffering from cancer. However, many of the issues discussed are common to any very sick child.

Parents who are told that their child is going to die have already been through a great deal of pain. They may have been dreading this moment on and off since their child's diagnosis, and will need help to come to terms with the fact that no matter how much more treatment their child is given, it will be to no avail.

Families of children with cancer live with constant uncertainty about the future, both during and after treatment. Worries about a relapse are often uppermost in their minds. In some instances the knowledge that a child's treatment is to be stopped, even though he is going to die, may actually be a relief to parents.

Acceptance of the change from curative treatment to palliative care is important both for the child's sake and the parent's eventual peace of mind. This is a big step and usually occurs gradually, rather than being an immediate change. A few families cannot contemplate the idea of their child receiving no further treatment, and following discussion with the medical staff a regime of therapy may be offered.

The initial reaction for many parents when told their child is going to die is to want to leave the hospital immediately and take their child home. It is the family's prerogative to choose where the child is cared for and where he is going to die. Although sometimes hard for us as professionals, the family must be helped to make the decision that is right for them, not the one which we feel most comfortable with. This is probably the most difficult and distressing time that a parent will ever have to face, so allowing time and space to make decisions is essential. Knowing that such decisions might be right for today but not for next week, and that they can be changed is important.

For many families the choice to be at home remains the right one, and with help and support from experienced professionals they can nurse their child at home until he dies. Some families want to be at home at first and then choose to take their child back into hospital, or a hospice, so that they do not feel isolated and frightened. They may even choose to take their child into hospital for the last few hours or days of his life. For some, nursing their child at home is what they wish to do, with frequent breaks at their local hospital or hospice. The extra support, peace of mind, and rest this gives them, may prove invaluable to the whole family.

Such respite from caring, especially in long ongoing situations, is important. Families should be aware from the outset that they do not have to be the primary carers all the time. Time for themselves and time to sleep is very important and benefits the child, as they will be rested and therefore more able to cope.

THE CARERS

There can be no question of the need for back-up and support for these families, but who is best placed to provide and coordinate this support?

Paediatric home care teams have evolved from the adult hospice movement, founded in 1967 by Dame Cicely Saunders. These services differ from those offered to adults who are terminally ill. A home care service is not only caring for the child but for his entire family, supporting and therefore enabling them to care for their child as long as they can. Children are not expected to die before their parents and grandparents. Support required may include help to alleviate the guilt felt by a grandparent for remaining alive while their young grandchild is dying.

Cancer, of which leukaemia is the most common type, is second to accidents in causing death in children aged 1–14 years [1]. This might suggest that a child dying of cancer is not a rare event. The fact is that cancer affects only one in 600 children in Britain and therefore most general practitioners would meet only one child suffering from cancer in their entire career. Today we expect 60–70% of these children to recover from their disease. Death among children suffering from other illnesses is even more uncommon, so it would be unrealistic to expect every general practitioner and primary health care team to become expert in the care of gravely ill and dying children.

It may well be that many of these children will not have seen their general practitioner during treatment as it will have been necessary for them to go directly to hospital if unwell. If a decision is made to care for the child at home their general practitioner will be actively involved as one of the prime carers.

Local primary health care teams, whose experience of a child dying, and therefore confidence in the situation, may be lacking, will value input from an expert source. Information regarding the location of specialist teams and their function(s) can be found in the Directory of Hospice Services [2].

The building up of a trusting relationship betwen the family and the professional will help all involved through the next few weeks and months. Some families may want regular visits or contact. Others will wish to remain very private and one should respect this and bear in mind that the professional is a visitor in the family home. It may be difficult for some to accept help initially as the mere fact that support is being offered reinforces the knowledge that their child is no longer curable. For the most effective support to be given the caring team must tailor their input accordingly.

Prior to the child's discharge for terminal care communication between the hospital and primary health care team is essential. The general practitioner is in a good position, in conjunction with the hospital liaison person, to assess the needs of the child and family. Initiating a meeting for all involved, including the family, will ensure that their needs are acknowledged. An identified key worker will facilitate care for the child and his family from this point thus enabling involvement of the appropriate professionals. Hopefully the family will then feel adequately supported but not overwhelmed.

The role of the professional will often be that of educating, encouraging and supporting, with the family wanting to deliver much of the care. Looking after a dying child is very different from nursing an adult in the last stages of life. Whereas a district nurse may well be required to help move or wash an immobile adult, a parent is often able to care for a child in this way with no assistance from the visiting professional. Indeed parents may resent such interference, which may be fulfilling a need of the professional rather than that of the family. A gentle reminder that help is available if required should ensure that families will ask for such help if they need it. Parents may change their minds from day to day, depending on many variables, not least because they are tired and under tremendous pressure. They may feel that while the situation remains as it is they can cope, but if the child becomes more sick or dependent they will no longer be able to. The child then deteriorates further, requiring the parents to develop new skills, and despite their worries they still manage this. Learning how to operate a subcutaneous syringe pump containing opiates is one example of the skills some parents acquire with remarkable speed. Many parents will choose to look after such a pump themselves rather than have to wait for a visit at uncertain times each day.

To avoid confusion, information given to the family must be consistent, and effective communication between carers will ensure this. Families in this situation will often ask the same questions time and time again and if given the same answers by each professional they will feel reassured that what they are doing is right.

FROM ACTIVE TO PALLIATIVE CARE

When the focus of care becomes palliative, the need for visits to the hospital may be reduced. For most families this gives rise to mixed emotions. While the idea of not having to journey backwards and forwards to hospital, and the wait to be seen each time, may be appealing, the idea of being separated from a safe environment, which has at times felt like a second home, is very frightening.

Decisions about follow-up will be dependent upon numerous variables. These include the wishes and needs of the family and the confidence in, and availability of, local resources. Parents are encouraged to feel that the option is always there should the family or carers ever feel that a hospital visit would be beneficial for further advice or information. A decision not to attend for regular clinic visits is likely to promote questions from the child and siblings as it is a sign that something has changed. This may give rise to questions which parents are not yet ready to deal with and should be taken into consideration when helping parents make such decisions.

BLOOD TRANSFUSIONS AND BLEEDING PROBLEMS

Throughout treatment patients and parents may have become used to having therapy based upon results; that is, when the child's platelet count or haemoglobin is low he will have received a transfusion. This makes it difficult for a parent or indeed a professional to feel confident in observation rather than scientific results.

During terminal care the ideal is to be as non-invasive as possible. In many cases it is possible to assess the need for blood and platelet transfusions by observation of symptoms rather than routine blood testing. However, worries about bleeding or breathlessness can conjure up very graphic pictures in the minds of parents and carers and for some this is unbearable. Some patients suffer from diseases which by their nature give rise to obvious bleeding problems. These would be groups of patients that one would test and transfuse regularly. For a small number of children bleeding will continue to be a problem despite regular platelet transfusions. The families of these children should be warned that it is possible that their child may go on to have a large bleed or even bleed to death.

Most parents will cope better, as new symptoms arise, if they have some prior knowledge and have been taught appropriate skills. Caring for a child who is drowsy, unconscious or even having convulsions, following a cerebral haemorrhage, will be very different from the distressing experience of a child who is having an uncontrollable bleed. Ensuring that the child's distress is relieved, by the use of sedation, is the most appropriate treatment. For a parent to know that the child is unaware may be comforting in this particular situation.

Most children with acute lymphoblastic leukaemia do not have bleeding problems even though many do have petechiae and some bruising.

Some parents may have vivid memories of other children who have had dramatic problems. While the family should be discouraged from making such comparisons, regular blood testing may be necessary for their peace of mind, although full blood counts do not always indicate how the child is. For example, a rising white cell and blast count may not have a direct relationship with the child's physical condition nor be guaranteed to give an idea of remaining lifespan. A blood transfusion may well provide good relief if a child is suffering symptoms of anaemia. If the sleepiness and lethargy are unresolved following transfusion, these symptoms may be due to disease progression. It may not, therefore, be appropriate to transfuse again.

NEEDLE PHOBIA

Needle phobia may be an issue and must be taken into consideration. Such a phobia could dictate the route by which symptomatic treatment is delivered.

Should any invasive procedure be necessary it is important to use the same techniques that proved useful during treatment so as to limit trauma to the child. These may include the use of local anaesthetic cream for venepuncture, setting up a subcutaneous infusion and even finger pricks, hypnotherapy and distraction techniques using bubble blowing, stories and puppets [3].

Families will need to be encouraged not to promise a child that there will be no more needles. This assumption that needles stop as treatment stops can be a very positive thought for a family at a time when all else seems to be negative. It can also create problems at a later stage. Children may go on to require subcutaneous drugs should they suffer from nausea, vomiting or become too sleepy to take their analgesic.

CENTRAL VENOUS ACCESS

If a child has a central line it will be used in preference to any other parenteral route. A central line is an indwelling catheter which provides constant venous access. It will most commonly be either a Hickman line (see Figure 10.1) or a Portacath. Whereas a Hickman line has an external catheter a Portacath consists of a subcutaneous reservoir. Both are inserted under general anaesthetic and can remain *in situ* throughout the course of the child's illness.

Even in situations when infusions of analgesia are necessary one would not suggest a subcutaneous route if such a line was available. In some situations a child may be considered a candidate for a new central line depending upon his disease and anticipated symptoms.

Maintenance care of these lines will be instigated by the child's treatment centre, who would always be willing to offer advice or

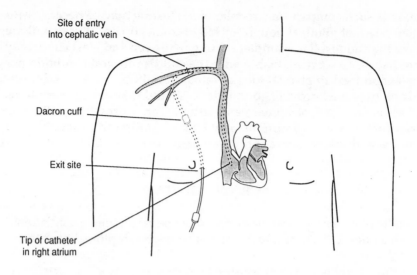

Site of entry
into cephalic vein

Dacron cuff

Exit site

Tip of catheter
in right atrium

Fig 10.1 A Hickman line

help to professionals working in the community. The line should be accessed using an aseptic technique and flushed regularly to ensure patency. Following teaching and supervision the parents or even the child may choose to care for the central line themselves.

ALTERNATIVE THERAPIES

For some families there is a great need to explore every possible treatment alternative. Options such as homeopathy, herbal medicine and faith healing can enable parents to know that they have tried everything available. Indeed these methods can also be used in conjunction with conventional medicine. As long as taking this avenue does not subject a sick child to countless trips around the country or unpleasant techniques and the cost to the family is reasonable, they need not be discouraged. Knowing they have explored these options may help later during the grieving process.

NUTRITION AND HYDRATION

Professionals are able to acknowledge that a dying child will increasingly lose his appetite as he deteriorates but it is part of the parenting role to feed and nourish a child. It is therefore understandable that for many parents it is a very difficult aspect of caring for their critically ill child. Many children, during treatment, will have had periods of anorexia and may have required parenteral feeding. This is hard enough to accept, despite its being a by-product of curative treatment. Even more difficult is the question of parenteral feeding in a palliative care setting. It is common for children to get increasingly anorexic as they become more unwell, many children eventually taking very little to eat or drink at all. Giving the parents encouragement to allow the child what he fancies when he asks is helpful but does not reduce the anxiety experienced by some families that their child might die more quickly without sufficient nourishment or fluid. The child's intake, oral or nasogastric, will also be dependent upon other symptoms. A child who is experiencing a sore mouth, constipation, nausea or vomiting, will obviously be less able to take food and fluids. There may be some improvement in intake and appetite with appropriate management of the problem.

NASOGASTRIC TUBE FEEDING

Some families will at this point question the place of nasogastric feeding. Although we can appreciate how difficult it is for parents to watch their child deteriorate in this way, as professionals the contra-indications to initiating feeding may be more obvious to us. These include, the unpleasant sensation of having a tube passed and kept in place, possible exacerbation of symptoms such as nausea and vomiting, and bringing the hospital equipment into the home environment. There are those children for whom nasogastric tube feeding is appropriate. A child with slow disease progression who is unable to drink or one who is uncomfortable due to fluid depletion may benefit from hydration until he deteriorates further.

If nasogastric or intravenous feeding is already established, it is more difficult to decide if and when to stop. Any change should be dependent upon how ready and prepared the family are at this stage. It may be that a gradual change in emphasis from a set feeding pattern to feeds at family meal time for example would allow time for adjustment. Frank discussion about a child's condition and deterioration is something that many parents value and expect from the professional. While it is difficult to anticipate exactly when a child will die, indicating that he is more poorly than the previous day, for example, will help a family appreciate that the child is nearer to death. It may be obvious to the professional that a child who has Cheyne–Stokes breathing is about to die, but a parent who has never seen anyone dying before will require constant explanation and support.

ALTERED BODY IMAGE

A reduction in oral intake will almost certainly result in weight loss. In some cases this can alter the child's appearance dramatically. This can also be an indication for tube feeding or dietary supplements, particularly for children with slowly progressive diseases. The appearance of the child is of great importance to those who love them. In any event the wishes of the parent must be paramount. It is not only parents who are affected by these physical changes but the child himself. An older child may be embarrassed or feel ugly. He may have changed physically due to his disease or treatment and this will have been difficult enough to cope with. Watching these gradual but sometimes dramatic changes of weight and muscle wasting can be unbearably distressing.

MOUTH CARE

As a child deteriorates, so will the condition of his mouth. The unpleasant sensations experienced due to problems such as dryness, halitosis, bleeding, candida or even ulceration can significantly add to how unwell a child feels.

Basic mouth care may prevent such problems occurring and, if the child allows, should be performed regularly. The use of a soft toothbrush may make teeth cleaning more bearable if the gums are sensitive. For a child who is either too upset, or non-compliant, even mouthwashes using water are preferable in order to keep the mouth clean. Practical hints on how parents can help their child feel more refreshed with flavoured ice cubes or lemon and glycerine mouth swabs may help, especially if the child's intake is minimal. Dry lips can be helped with vaseline or the pleasantly flavoured lip balms produced commercially.

CONSTIPATION

Constipation is a common problem and may be due to lack of fluids, poor food intake, lack of muscle tone, lack of mobility, or the use of opiates.

Use of an appropriate toilet, bedpan or commode on which the child feels comfortable and safe can be a help. Ensure privacy wherever possible. Diet and fluid advice, warm drinks, and even cuddling a hot water bottle may help. It is important to monitor bowel function carefully, as constipation can result in distressing symptoms.

URINARY SYMPTOMS

Check for infection. A urinary tract infection can be particularly painful and distressing, and even if the child is very poorly this type of infection should be treated with antibiotics as this is the most appropriate way to alleviate this particular pain.

A warm bath or the sound of running taps may help a child to pass urine. As a last resort catheterization with a small size catheter may be necessary.

LOSS OF BODY FUNCTION

Not only having to cope with the fact that he is going to die from his disease but also a loss of body function when he is still relatively well is yet another insult. A child who can no longer climb the stairs and is too heavy to carry may find it humiliating to have his bed moved downstairs or even to have to use a commode. Being dependent on someone else for help with ordinary tasks is likely to make anyone feel vulnerable. Becoming incontinent can mean that an older child feels that he has regressed to being a baby. To be reliant upon carers for such basic needs can result in a total loss of dignity. Even a child who is recently potty trained could find reverting to nappies very upsetting.

Dying children may spend their last few days or weeks alternating between being relatively well and able to do some of their favourite things, and feeling tired and sleeping for many hours each day. Parents need to be aware that this is not uncommon, thus enabling them to continue to appreciate that their child is dying. Changes in condition may be due to adjustments in medication. For instance, if he is given appropriate analgesia, a child who was previously in pain will be more willing to move around. Encouraging everyone to make the most of a child's well periods is important as gradually the good days will decrease and the sleepiness and general deterioration become more apparent.

A change of toys may be necessary to enable this so that the child can be kept occupied during his alert moments. Reading books, listening to tapes and videos are invaluable for children of all ages.

FITTING

As professionals who encourage honesty within the family we must be honest with them ourselves. By telling them what we think and feel about their child's condition we can perhaps give some indication about the progression of their child's disease. Telling parents that their child may have a fit, for example, can be frightening. Explaining to them what it might be like and leaving appropriate medications and instructions in the house will mean that if the situation arises, parents may feel less frightened and more confident.

SKIN CARE

Many of the children have very fragile skin, particularly if they have been on steroids, have striae or are very thin or obese.

If a child is no longer able to move around by himself and is spending more time sitting in a chair and lying in bed, he will be vulnerable to developing pressure sores and special attention must be given to the condition of his skin. Bruising may also be a problem for some children and providing the family with a Spenco, a ripple mattress or sheepskin, and ensuring they are aware of the importance of changing his position at regular intervals, will be beneficial. Adequate control of the child's pain is essential for this to be possible. A child experiencing pain will find even the slightest movements more difficult. Some children may be more comfortable in an electric bed, or may find being moved in a hoist less traumatic.

Itchiness of the skin can be a problem for some children who suffer from metabolic or liver disorders. The use of diamorphine can also cause an itchiness. Cool baths, a cool atmosphere and cotton clothing may all help. Creams or oils may help a dry skin.

OEDEMA OF HANDS AND FEET

Elevation of limbs on pillows will help, as will massaging of the affected hands or feet with nice smelling aromatherapy oils. This can be a soothing and pleasant experience for the child, and for the parent, grandparent or sibling who is doing the massaging.

USEFUL AIDS TO OFFER AT HOME

A baby alarm may help to keep parents in touch with what is happening in the child's room, particularly at night time, and allows the child the security of being able to call for help. A wheelchair or buggy increases opportunities to go outside. A hoist may be a help for children who are heavy or awkward to lift. A backrest, extra pillows, Spenco mattress, sheepskin and bedcradle may all help with comfort in bed. A bedpan, a urine bottle, a commode and incontinence pads may be necessary. A fan may help to keep a child comfortable.

A telephone answering machine may give periods of relief from an endless barrage of well-meaning enquiries.

TALKING AND LISTENING

When a child is dying, parents will have endless questions, worries and fears for which they will need answers and explanations. One of the most common questions asked by parents is 'how long?' They may be given an approximate range, i.e. weeks not months, months not years. This information will be based upon the child's condition, and past experience with certain diseases. Although it is possible to give an idea of the length of time anticipated, it is unwise to do more than this as even this is often difficult to assess.

Some families may choose to take their child on holiday and will often ask advice from professionals. If the trip is important to them and the child is well enough, they should not be discouraged. However, they need to be aware that the child may become unwell or die while away. Discussing such issues as medical insurance, which can be difficult to obtain as well as expensive, early flights home or even bringing a child's body home after has has died, will help them to make a decision. For some families the fear is too great and they choose to remain at home.

'Why our child?' is a question asked by many families at some stage of their child's terminal illness. There can be no explanation of course, but simply by listening the professional can help to untangle the confusion felt by many parents in this situation.

The opportunity to discuss their worries, changes in the child's condition and any new problems should be available 24 hours a day. The family may not feel able to talk about sensitive issues at the time of a home visit, but require answers and explanations at other times.

Talking to the dying child and his brothers and sisters is a subject which parents will often want advice about. Depending upon the ages of the children and their parents' beliefs, there are many ways to prepare children for what lies ahead. Encouraging families to be honest and to try to answer their children's questions as simply and truthfully as possible, will help them to understand what is happening. Knowing what is real is far less frightening to a young child than allowing his imagination to run away with him. He may conjure up all sorts of frightening and vivid thoughts in his mind, when often a simple explanation could avoid such fear and upset. Telling a child that his brother or sister has gone to sleep, for example, may cause sleepless nights as the child fears the same may happen to him.

Many parents feel that they cannot cope with talking to their dying child about his own death. This attitude can be difficult for a professional whose experience will demonstrate the benefits of an open approach. For example, if a child is not given the opportunity to express his feelings and wishes, he may be anxious, worried or depressed, and may also be deprived of time to finish things off. Writing a will, celebrating a birthday or buying and wrapping Christmas presents may be very important to him. For the parents and siblings encouragement to take photographs or even video film of the child can provide enjoyment now and some comfort after the child's death.

It is never possible to prepare parents fully for the death of a child but visiting regularly and anticipating changes will enable the professional to discuss parents' worries and fears with them as they arise. Some families will need reassuring that someone will visit when death seems imminent while other families will prefer to be left alone with their child.

CARE OF THE UNCONSCIOUS CHILD

The anxiety of the parents about feeding their child may increase at this stage. Encourage them to continue to keep the child's mouth moist and fresh and re-assure them that the child is very unlikely to be feeling hungry. Encourage the parents to continue to touch or cuddle their child, and to continue to talk to him.

TIME OF DEATH

If families are prepared for what may happen then they will be less worried. Changes of colour and cold extremities can be very worrying if parents have not been warned that these changes are very common. Some parents have been very distressed that their child 'became incontinent' at the time of death, and also worried by 'bruising' which appears soon after death and is caused by settling of the blood. Simple explanations beforehand can avoid unnecessary distress. Explain what is happening if parents hear a 'death rattle' or Cheyne–Stokes respirations. The sighing sound which a child may make if he is moved soon after death does not mean that he is still alive.

AFTER DEATH

Once the child has died it is important that the parents are aware that there is no urgency for the body to be removed. It is acceptable to spend time with their dead child if they wish. There may be practices that are stipulated within specific faiths that do not allow such flexibility and the professional must be aware of these differences [4]. Parents will require reassurance that they can still hold their child. They may want to take a photograph, or invite family and friends to come to the house and say their goodbyes. The may wish to wash him and dress him in his favourite clothes and perhaps put a special teddy or toy with his body before it is taken away.

Before any practical arrangements can be carried out, a doctor must certify the child as dead. There is no urgency for this although the doctor must have seen the child during the previous two weeks in order to sign the certificate and prevent the need to report the death to the coroner and possible necessity of a post-mortem.

Making decisions immediately after the child's death can be so difficult that arrangements may be left to the undertakers. Talking to the undertakers prior to the death will have provided the family with an opportunity to discuss preferences about embalming, make up, removal of lines or catheters as well as the more obvious points like the costs of the funeral.

For most parents the physical removal of their child's body from the house is extremely distressing. Indeed some families will choose to keep their child at home until the funeral.

Once the body has been taken from the house the parents can arrange with the undertakers to visit the chapel of rest and see their child before the funeral. They may choose to take brothers and sisters and other relatives especially if the child looks peaceful. Parents will often ask for advice regarding brothers and sisters attending the funeral. With this, as with every other issue, decisions should be made with the individual's interests and wishes foremost. The type of service that parents want for their child is again something that may have been talked about before the child has died [5]. Decisions about a burial or cremation and what they wish to do with their child's ashes, are often easier to make while the child is still alive. If parents have particular religious beliefs they may want to discuss their wishes with their local clergyman. Their faith may already have been of great support and will perhaps be invaluable in the months that lie ahead. For some families religion does not figure in their lives and a personal service run entirely without any religious input at their local crematorium, or elsewhere, may be what they choose. Parents may wish to incorporate a favourite story or piece of music into the service. It is generally possible to accommmodate the wishes of any family whether traditional or otherwise.

Families wishing to bury their child abroad will require the assistance and experience of the undertaker who is usually willing to help the family as much as possible, and if told of the parents' wishes and desires will ensure that these are carried out to the best of his ability.

While concentrating on caring for the child in his own home, this chapter touches briefly on many aspects of death in childhood. In any practical sense it is difficult if not impossible to separate care into discrete categories. It is essential to take into account not only the child but the physical, psychological and emotional needs of the whole family, each member of the family having individual feelings.

As carers we must remember that what seems right for us is not always right for a family. We should try to be aware of our prejudices and not impress our own views and ideals upon them. Hopefully decisions will be made in partnership with the family to ensure the best possible care for the child and in order that the family have no regrets about the care their child received.

Individual professionals may not feel confident looking after a dying child even though they may have looked after terminally ill adults. Advice and information from an expert source can prove invaluable. Availability of resources varies from area to area. Knowing what is available locally and using resources appropriately will ensure that the child and his family receive optimum care.

If home is the place of choice it should, ideally, remain a private environment where professional help is welcome and available whenever needed. Flexibility and open mindedness will help to ensure that, as far as possible, the restrictions of the hospital are not brought into the home. This should help the family to feel cocooned rather than overwhelmed by the professionals caring for their child. Whatever decisions the family makes, both before the death of their child and afterwards, will hopefully be right for them. The professional can only advise, and give support in the hope that the family will feel they have dealt with a difficult and distressing situation as best they could.

REFERENCES

1. Cancer Research Campaign (1990) Fact Sheet: Childhood Cancer UK. 15 January.
2. Directory of Hospice Services in the UK and Republic of Ireland (1991) Compiled by St Christopher's Hospice Information Service.
3. Lansdown, R. (1987) *Helping Children Cope with Needles. A Guide for Parents and Staff*, Department of Psychological Medicine, Great Ormond Street Hospital, London.
4. Green, J. (1991) *Death with Dignity – Meeting the Spiritual Needs of Patients in a Multi-cultural Society*. Nursing Times Publication, Macmillan, London.
5. Walter, Tony (1990) *Funerals and How to Improve Them*, Hodder and Stoughton, London.

CHAPTER 11

The role of the children's hospice

Lenore Hill

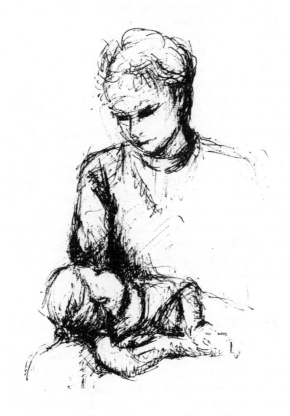

Hospice: A house of rest and entertainment for pilgrims, travellers or strangers.

Shorter Oxford Dictionary

THE BEGINNINGS

Helen House, the first hospice for sick children and their families in the United Kingdom, and probably the world, was opened in Oxford in 1982. The concept arose from the friendship of Mother Frances Dominica, the then Superior General of the Anglican Order of All Saints, with Helen and her family. Helen was a very sick little girl following surgery to remove a brain tumour. During Helen's long stay in hospital her baby sister was born. Mother Frances had no answers to the great emotional pain of the family but showed her willingness to be alongside them in their anguish, sharing their burden. In so doing she unconsciously established the foundation of the children's hospice philosophy.

It became obvious at an early stage of the friendship between Frances and Helen's parents that there was a physical as well as an emotional burden in caring for this very precious little girl. One weekend Frances asked permission to 'borrow' Helen and care for her in the convent. She undertook to care for her in the way that she was cared for at home. She kept to her timetable, chose her favourite foods, and sang her favourite nursery rhymes. After several such breaks, the idea of extending the friendship, help and support that Frances offered Helen and her parents to other families in similar situations emerged. The idea for Helen House was born.

The advice of Helen's parents and Mother Frances Dominica in the design and equipping of Helen House ensured the home-from-home atmosphere and friendly feel of the hospice. In particular, Helen's parents felt it was very important that the number of bedrooms should not exceed eight, because they felt that the individual nature and the quality of the care offered would be jeopardized if the hospice were on a larger scale.

The size and guiding philosophy of Helen House have been available as a model for those who have followed.

THE CHILDREN'S HOSPICE MOVEMENT

At the time of writing, 1992, there are five children's hospices open and several appeals for more are established. We do need more than the present number but it is important that they develop in areas that best serve the needs of the families. The number of children with life-threatening, life-limiting or terminal disorders is mercifully small. The current thinking is that we probably need one for each health region in England, and two each in Scotland and Wales. Certainly the five existing children's hospices are finding it increasingly difficult to provide adequate care for all the children referred to them.

Of these five children's hospices I only have intimate knowledge of the working of three, Helen House in Oxford, Francis House in

Manchester and Martin House in Clifford, Yorkshire. I believe that the philosophy of the other existing and projected hospices is likely to be much the same, although the methods of working may differ. Some have the active involvement of a religious order, and have a chapel available on site for the use of families. All have chaplains, and all welcome and make provision for families of any race, religion or culture.

WHO CAN USE A CHILDREN'S HOSPICE?

Any family who have a child or children with a life-threatening, life-limiting or terminal disorder can use a children's hospice. In practice this means that the majority of the children using these facilities suffer from progressive disorders such as the inborn errors of metabolism or neuromuscular degenerative diseases. There is a smaller but significant group with cancer, and a large miscellaneous group which includes children with cystic fibrosis, renal, liver and heart disease. Children with non-progressive handicap cannot normally be accepted unless the degree of handicap is so severe as to be, in itself, life-limiting.

WHO CAN REFER A CHILD TO A CHILDREN'S HOSPICE?

An appropriate referral will be accepted from anyone. Many requests for help come directly from families, or from family support groups. School teachers, social workers, other charities, health visitors and nurses as well as GPs and consultants all refer children.

Permission is always asked to contact the GP and the consultant for information and to ensure cooperation in care.

WHAT SERVICES ARE OFFERED?

The children's hospices do not see themselves as substitutes for good hospital or community care, and would indeed wish to identify with those seeking to achieve excellence of service in those areas for all families with sick or handicapped children.

Service and friendship

The care teams within the children's hospices include many with appropriate qualifications such as registered sick children's nurses, paediatric physiotherapists, teachers, social workers and nursery nurses. Nevertheless, although these skills may be useful to the families, the aim of all those on the team, with or without professional qualification, is to meet the families just as themselves. They offer friendship and service not professionalism and direction. To this end no one wears uniform, everyone is known by their first name, and families are expected and encouraged to be in control. Every attempt is made to match as nearly as possible the parental care patterns set at home. Members of the care team are in touch with the families regularly throughout the time of involvement, continuing this friend-ship into the families' own homes.

Flexible support

As far as resources allow, support is offered in as flexible a way as possible. For some families all that is asked is regular contact at home, with the knowledge that help, advice and support are at the end of a telephone at any time of the night or day. Support is offered to all members of the family and often the well children in the family, and the grandparents, need a listening ear and someone who will take their pain and problems seriously.

The birthdays of the well children are remembered as faithfully as those of the sick ones, and if treats or trips out are arranged, well siblings are always included. Some families, in times of acute difficulty, may need a service at home which is not currently available from community services. This is particularly so if 24-hour care is needed over short periods of time in order to keep the child at home.

Some families have been totally unaware of other resources available to them, and have needed advice and help to claim basic support such as attendance allowance and mobility allowance.

Some families have felt threatened by case conferences called to dis-cuss the 'failure to thrive' of a child suffering from a progressive disorder. The parents have requested support at such meetings from a member of the care team who, they feel, will understand the degenerative nature of the disease and the difficulties they may have in feeding their child.

Respite with the child

All of the families using the children's hospices want to care for their children themselves throughout the illness. For many that illness may involve a very prolonged period of watching their child's disease progress, the child becoming steadily more dependent and more difficult to care for physically and emotionally. Many parents really appreciate an opportunity to get away from the four walls of home, away from the duties of daily household chores, the demands of the telephone, and even, sometimes, of well-meaning friends or relatives. While in the hospice they can, if they wish, give up responsibility for changing dirty nappies, feeding, which may take 2 hours for one meal, and washing and ironing the clothes. They can still enjoy time cuddling or playing with their child, or spending time in the multisensory room or the jacuzzi. It is good for couples to be able to spend time talking and listening to each other, and doing 'normal' things such as playing, shopping or going on trips out with their well children.

Some families ask for the child to be cared for while they do something else altogether. It may be for only a few hours while the child's mother gets her hair done or goes shopping. It can be for up to two weeks to facilitate home decorations or a family holiday. Some adolescents prefer to come alone, appreciating the opportunity of some 'independence'.

We usually request that families stay with their children, at least on their first visit, so that we can get to know them as a family, and be sure that we have learnt to carry out care in the way that they would wish us to.

The children, sick or well, love to visit, and every effort is made to ensure that they enjoy their 'holidays' with us. Lots of busy activities, games, painting, model-making, as well as trips out to local places of interest and the cinema, will help to enhance the quality of life of these children.

Listening ears

Older children and adolescents whose disease has not caused neurological damage will often want to talk about their situation. Care team members need to have ears trained to pick up the cues, and to help the children to open areas of discussion which they may find difficult. Whatever they want to talk about must be accepted and heard in a non-judgemental way: what they feel is real to them and cannot be 'reasoned away'.

Many hours are also spent by members of the care team listening to parents as they talk through the pain of their situation and their plans, hopes and fears for the future. As has been said before, other members of the family will also need to be heard, as may teachers, school friends and other carers.

Parents can often be a great resource to other families and will spend many hours listening to each other. They can be a source of inspiration and of practical ideas. The care team can never say 'I know how you feel'; the families, to some extent, do have a shared experience.

Emergency respite

Domestic emergencies which may occur in any family can be a real crisis for the family where one child or more is sick. Wherever possible a hospice would accept a child for emergency respite care where another child or parent is sick, or some other household emergency arises.

Symptom control

Throughout the course of many progressive disorders new features arise necessitating a change in medical and nursing management. Examples of this include seizures and the need to start anti-convulsants, increased secretions or poor swallowing necessitating the consideration of tube feeding. Sometimes it is appropriate for the child to be hospitalized until the new management is established. More often this can be achieved at home if enough support is available. Some parents prefer the support to be offered within the relaxed environment of the hospice.

Terminal care

If at all possible terminal care should be offered wherever the child and the family wish for death to take place. The children sometimes die very suddenly and unexpectedly, or in the middle of some acute episode which has necessitated hospitalization. Some children and parents feel safe in a ward among familiar staff who may have treated the child frequently over the years of the illness.

Most of our parents would choose death at home, but several want a member of the hospice staff to be with them for the last few days of their child's life. For many families this is their first experience of death, and they appreciate the presence of someone who has the experience they lack.

A significant number of people choose the hospice as the place of death for their child. The reasons are probably as varied as the people. Some parents feel that they would not be able to continue to live in their present home if their child had died there. Some appreciate the fact that, although they can have as much privacy as they want, and can stay in control of decisions and choices, there is plenty of support and company around immediately they want to use it. There is also support there for the well children, who can have as much involvement with their dying sibling as they wish, but can, when they prefer, join in other activities within the house. Other responsibilities of daily life are removed, allowing quality time together with the sick child.

There is a big comfortable double bed which the dying child can share with parents, siblings and pets as desired. There is no rush and as much time as is wanted can be spent with the child at the time of death and in the days before the funeral.

The cold bedroom

A facility is provided which looks like a bedroom, but can be chilled down to keep a child's body cold. After the parents have washed and dressed the child, and whenever they are ready to do so the child is carried to this room. He is placed in a bed or cot, with a favourite duvet cover and favourite toys. Many other items may be placed in the room by families. These are as various as religious symbols, flowers, football scarves and firemen's helmets. The family has unrestricted access and can pick up the child, or talk to him for as long as they wish, although for some families this available time is constrained by religious beliefs. For most this gives plenty of time for 'goodbyes', easy access for siblings in a non-threatening environment, and time to complete plans for the funeral, cremation or burial without being hurried. Where the death of their child has taken place either in hospital or at home an increasing number of families are wanting to use the facility of this cold bedroom for the days between the death and the funeral. The whole family usually stays in the hospice for this time.

Bereavement support

Current experience of the hospices seems to indicate that regular support is needed for two to three years following the death of a child. When regular visiting stops, by mutual agreement with the family, they are always left with the telephone number and the invitation to ring in the future if they need someone to talk to. Times that would have been landmarks for the child, in his school life or special family occasions, can suddenly cause great pain. Anniversaries of the birth and death are remembered and shared with the family for the first few years. Special times for the family, such as setting of headstones, are times which they will often ask the care team to share with them.

Once a year the hospice holds a service of remembrance and thanksgiving for the lives of the children who have died, and the whole day is set aside for bereaved families. This gives them an opportunity to come back to a place which is often special to them in the memories they have of their child.

A HOME FROM HOME

The size, the design, the furnishings and the staffing of the children's hospices are all intended to create a home-from-home environment. The hospices are purposely small: the current ones have between seven and ten beds for sick children. They have lots of accommodation for parents and siblings, as well as pets. The main living accommodation is fairly open plan, with the kitchen being central to life, as it is in most homes. (Most children love to bake.)

Although each facility is small, the number of families being supported by the individual hospices varies from 120 to 200 at any one time, plus large numbers of bereaved families. The children's hospice should be seen as just one resource available to hard-pressed families trying to achieve the best care possible for their children during their short lives.

CHAPTER 12

Perinatal death

Elizabeth Hopper

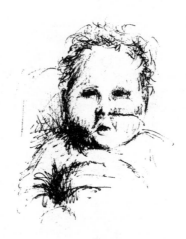

INTRODUCTION

The pain and fear of death makes it difficult to mention, except perhaps in hushed tones behind closed doors, and briefly, lest in some mysterious way it may creep towards us. And yet most would acknowledge the profound effect the death of a loved one has and the intense feelings that can be aroused. This is no less true for the death of a baby, whether before or after its birth.

'It was as if the birds would never sing again': Grace, now in her seventies, being interviewed, recalls the morning the doctor came into her room with those dreaded words: 'Your baby died this morning, about an hour ago. We tried . . .' [1] and his voice trailed away. Fifty years on and Grace still cries as she remembers Louise and her short life. Health professionals could learn much from listening to Grace's story, and the powerful effects of a miscarriage, a stillbirth and a neonatal death on her life, and that of her partner, Henry, and inevitably their families.

In this chapter the story of Grace and Henry, as well as more recent experiences of couples who babies have died, will be drawn upon together with reference to current literature which might help us see how such families may be cared for most appropriately. Following an overview, six headings are used to explore this: prenatal loss; neonatal death; follow-up care; the family; the next pregnancy; and the health professionals.

AN OVERVIEW

In recent years there has been more acknowledgement of the impact of the loss of life before birth and this has led to some changes in practice, both in hospital and community settings. What seems to be particularly interesting, however, is that despite 20 years and more of research evidence to suggest preferable ways of caring for women and their partners suffering perinatal loss, there is still much that needs serious attention in such a sensitive area.

At a time of rapid change, including considerable technological advances, both in obstetrics and paediatrics, it is remarkable that so little consideration is being given to the psychological implications of these developments. For now, not only are there many lay people who consider the gestational age of viability to have dropped so low that if some babies survive being born at 23 weeks' gestation, then probably theirs will, but also others who hope that even that gestational limit will be surpassed as technology advances. It is important to note, I believe, that the more the expectations of good outcome in pregnancy are heightened, the harder still we will find it to talk of endings and death.

Of course, no one would wish to return to the days of high perinatal mortality, and yet when death was less of a taboo, perhaps there was also a greater access to certain rituals and ways of dealing with grief and mourning. This is certainly true for many people in different parts of the world today. The paucity of our language and ways of dealing with death, especially the death of a child, makes it all the more difficult when problems, and therefore the prospect of poor outcome, are evident.

The way in which women with so called 'high risk pregnancies' are cared for in the antenatal period will be of utmost importance in terms not only of how they cope with the course of their pregnancy, but also its outcome.

PRENATAL LOSS

Borg and Lasker, in their book *When Pregnancy Fails*, quote a psychiatrist: 'Miscarriages do not occur in a uterus but in a woman, and miscarriages do not occur solely in a woman but in a family [2].

Grace was pregnant for the first time when, she recalls:

I began to haemorrhage. It was about my third month. I was in real trouble – very heavy bleeding. Even before I got to the hospital I knew I had lost the baby. Henry called for an ambulance. At the hospital they took me to surgery and did a D & C, which supposedly ended the episode. I was disappointed. I felt I had let Henry down and began to wonder what I might have done to bring on the miscarriage. Everyone . . . kept trying to reassure me that everything was just fine and that I could always have another baby. I was not so sure about what I was hearing them say. [1]

It is well known amongst health professionals working in accident and emergency, obstetrics, gynaecology and midwifery that miscarriage in the first trimester of pregnancy is common: around one in four pregnancies ends this way. For the woman miscarrying, it can be a frightening and often painful experience. It may be her first pregnancy or her fourth. She may have no children or several. She may have had 12 years of infertility and this was an *in vitro* fertilization (IVF) pregnancy. Whatever it has been, a woman's obstetric history is both important and relevant. Her reaction, and that of her partner and family, will be better understood and met if that history is known and acknowledged.

Caroline, who had had extensive investigations and lengthy fertility treatment, was eventually pregnant after 10 years. When she began to bleed in the ninth week of her pregnancy she was devastated. She arrived in casualty crying out 'Please don't let my baby die!' and was told to 'Pull herself together, she was only nine weeks pregnant'. These terse remarks from a busy Sister have stayed with Caroline for years after the event. David Cummings, writing about 'The effects of miscarriage on a man', recalls:

After checking on my wife and knowing that she was all right, I broke down and cried. All my dreams and hopes were gone. It was as if someone had stolen something very close to me. As I waited for my wife to recover, I kept wondering how and why something like this could happen. No one could answer my questions. We waited the six weeks and the doctors said no abnormalities were found. It was just one of those things as far as they could tell [3].

We can be sure that each loss will have its particular significance for a couple, especially if there is a history of infertility or recurrent miscarriage. While a miscarriage in early pregnancy is different from the loss of a baby later in pregnancy, there are, however, similarities that should not be overlooked. When a couple first know a pregnancy is definite, there is often a mixture of feelings. Whatever those feelings, what is inescapable to a greater or lesser extent, is that there will be hopes, dreams and expectations. When a pregnancy ends in tragedy the future has been changed and adjustments will need to be made according to the amount invested in the anticipated baby; that investment is likely to grow as the pregnancy progresses. Family, friends and professionals all ask about the baby. As movements begin and it becomes increasingly obvious to everyone that a baby is due, it is likely that parental attachment to the baby grows. It cannot simply be assumed however that the larger the baby in utero, the greater the sense of loss when the baby dies. The grief experienced may be much more related to the emotional investment made by parents, grand-parents and siblings.

The mother who has felt her baby moving and kicking inside her has experienced a unique relationship of intimacy. No one has known the baby as she has. The particular difficulty she may encounter if she is told there is a problem with the baby (an abnormality, life-threatening condition or death), is that she will be faced with grieving for a part of herself. She has not known the baby as a separate being. As Grubb-Phillips writes 'She has to cut short the normal processes of attachment and objectification and substitute the process of bereavement' [4]. This sudden change in direction takes some time of adjustment. Families will be assisted with this if they can be helped to understand some of the grieving processes, and they will be reassured to learn that others have shared similar feelings. In this respect, the part played by self-help groups is of crucial importance.

Sarah, after attending the local Stillbirth and Neonatal Death Society (SANDS) group for the first time, said 'I had no idea that other people felt as I do. It was such a relief to listen to other people. I began to feel I was normal after all, and that maybe things would get better.' Parents will be most helped by being put in touch with the group best suited to their needs. The Miscarriage Association, who have published 'Guidelines for Good Practice' [5] aimed at health professionals, gives specific help to women who lose a baby earlier in pregnancy. Women who experience recurrent miscarriage particularly have found great comfort in being known and supported by a group of women who meet regularly in each others' homes. Partners also are invited and can discover it to be a relief to find there are other men going through similar difficulties.

Support after Termination for Abnormality (SATFA) is another parent self-help group. They have produced a booklet [6] to be given to parents at the time of diagnosis of an abnormality. It outlines all the areas to be considered in contemplating termination, as well as offering continued support after the decision is made.

SANDS have also produced some literature. Their 'Guidelines for Professionals' [7] gives comprehensive details of caring for parents and families. They also provide a booklet, 'Saying Goodbye to Your Baby', which should be available to parents who experience a loss from around 20 weeks' gestation.

When Grace was of childbearing age in the 1930s there was no such system of support. She recalls after losing a stillborn baby she never saw:

> When I came home, we just didn't know what to do. Twice I had expected to come home with a baby. So we just gathered up all those baby things, put them on the mattress and covered the whole thing up with a bed sheet. We shoved everything back into a corner [1].

In 'Guidelines for Professionals', it is suggested:

Parents may want to:

- Wash their baby, or help, or watch this being done.
- Dress their baby in special clothes.
- Collect mementoes of their baby, such as a lock of hair, foot and hand prints, the cot card, weight and measurements, and so on.
- Take photos before and after death, and with the family if wanted.
- Put a small toy or something else that is personally significant into the moses basket with their baby.
- Ask the hospital chaplain or their own minister to give a blessing or say prayers for their baby.
- Take their baby home for a while, or keep the baby at home and make their own funeral arrangements.

As has already been mentioned, there have been changes in practice in recent years. It is no longer appropriate to discourage parents from seeing their baby, at any gestation, and even with an abnormality. Although of course the wishes of each individual must be respected, especially when these relate to religious or cultural observances, many parents have been grateful to have been, very gently, encouraged to see their baby even when they have been initially adamant they would rather not. In *When Pregnancy Fails*, Borg and Lasker write:

> Often when parents do not see their dead infant, they imagine him or her as being terribly deformed or ugly. Seeing the baby is a relief to many. If the baby is deformed, it is helpful to have the midwife explain to the parents what the defects are so that

they will know what to expect ... Most parents focus on features, even when the baby does not look normal. They tend to remember characteristics that resemble family members and to think of the baby as beautiful [2].

NEONATAL DEATH

Louise was such a beautiful baby girl. I wanted her so badly. And to have carried her all those months, having her those first few days, holding her, loving her and then, to have her get so sick all of a sudden and to die. It was so unfair. I still remember her birthday [1].

Grace recalled vividly, and tearfully her own story of losing her baby after a full-term pregnancy. For parents, memories of their baby's birth, brief life and death will last a lifetime. Good support given at the time could prevent future difficulties, for instance, pathological grief responses and other psychiatric sequelae. Health professionals have a crucial part to play when a baby is known to be dying as well as in the months and years after the baby's death.

Having a baby in a Neonatal or Special Care Baby Unit inevitably causes parents some concern. If the stay is fairly brief and good progress is maintained, parents may feel less anxious than when there is a long uncertain future ahead.

If a baby is becoming so unwell that the health professionals are aware that it is most unlikely the baby will survive, the parents should be informed immediately and preferably together. When there is a delay in giving parents the choice to be involved at this stage, they can be haunted by lifelong regrets.

Breaking bad news

Breaking bad news is never easy, but the very act is an opportunity to assist parents to begin the painful process of grieving well.

It is clear that some parents will want to know more details than others about their child's condition. However, even when questions are not being asked, professionals should be offering explanations if there is serious concern for the baby. Anxiety and fear sometimes paralyse parents so that they find it hard to know what to say. To be plunged into such an extraordinary environment of machinery, alarms, heat, and hand washing can be extremely daunting, especially if it is also experienced after a Caesarean section.

Angelina experienced just this. At 20 years of age, in her first pregnancy, she arrived at the hospital in labour. The baby was distressed, needed to be delivered by Caesarean section, and was then transferred to the Neonatal Unit. Angelina was taken to see the baby once she had recovered from the anaesthetic. Her reaction during the first few days appeared to indicate she wanted little to do with the baby or the doctors and nurses caring for him. She asked no questions, and showed little interest, even when his condition worsened. One particular nurse took time to explain what was happening with the baby each day. On the fifth day, when Angelina began to feel physically better, she confided to the nurse that she had begun, but not completed, training as a nursery nurse. This had been her nightmare, to have a very sick newborn. However, slowly Simon's condition improved and Angelina felt able to participate more in his care. The nurse's sensitivity and insight enabled Angelina to feel involved, while at the same time her own need for space was respected.

If a woman is physically unwell herself following birth, it is not unusual for her to find it difficult to concentrate on her baby whether or not the baby is sick or preterm. A mother in these circumstances requires care, and should not be made to feel guilty if she can take only scant interest in her baby while she is recovering herself.

Often the prognosis for a baby is uncertain. Parents find it easier if they have one professional to whom they can turn for comprehensive information about their baby. That person needs to be available for questions, and this will necessitate good communication between the staff involved to know when, how and by whom the information can be conveyed.

As soon as the prognosis is clear and the baby is unlikely to survive, parents need to be involved in the decision-making. The full implications of discontinuing active treatment and why that is being considered need to be explained to the parents.

Even when parents are aware that their baby's condition has been deteriorating, it will still come as a shock to talk of stopping treatment. This needs to be done carefully and gently, again preferably by a health professional they have come to know and trust.

Wherever possible the parents should be offered privacy but not be isolated or abandoned. It is likely that they have not seen anyone die before, and they may not feel able to say they are afraid. Health professionals will need to be alert to particular concerns. Where there is uncertainty whether to stay with parents or leave them alone together with the baby, asking what they prefer can avoid awkwardness and the making of inaccurate assumptions.

The particular difficulty of a baby dying at a very early age is that the parents have so little time to say their 'hellos' before they are preparing for 'goodbye'. It is appropriate therefore to give full attention to parental wishes as well as giving information about choices available to them. These should include those outlined above in the SANDS recommendations.

In addition, if a baby has been intensively nursed and has had several tubes of various kinds, these should be removed so that the parents can cuddle their baby with the possibility of maximum skin-to-skin contact.

If the hospital has a bereavement officer, she or he may be the person to liaise between different people on behalf of the parents, and also help to bridge the gap between hospital and community.

Parents should never feel hurried in their goodbyes either with their baby, or with the staff. There are certain practicalities that need attention at this time, but perhaps just as important as ensuring these are attended to is giving the space each parent needs to grieve in their own way. Sensitive support given at this stage may save parents and other family members much heartache in the months and years to come. Helping to provide parents and families with positive lasting memories will mean considerably enhanced prospects for a healthy grieving period and more resolved future.

Faiths and funerals

It is wise for health professionals not to make assumptions about parents' religious beliefs, values or practices based on what is entered on the mother's notes. For example, it may be that at the booking clinic, a woman said 'none' to the question of religion, but at a time of crisis may find comfort in seeing a religious adviser from her own cultural background. This is a sensitive area, and professionals should ask parents what they need and help them to make contact with the appropriate person. This may be a hospital chaplain or representative from their own religion in the community. The local Community Health Council or Community Relations Council may be able to help with this. Ensuring the baby is baptised, blessed or prayed for in the tradition the parents wish is the health professional's responsibility.

Hospital chaplains can be a source of comfort for parents of any religion or none. When parents feel ready to discuss possibilities for a funeral, chaplains can give information relevant to their hospital practices. Many hospitals offer a simple burial or cremation free of charge. If parents wish to arrange a funeral themselves, a list of funeral directors, cemetery and crematorium authorities should be made available. Details of the registration process for the baby's birth and death also need to be explained.

FOLLOW-UP CARE

A senior member of either the obstetric or paediatric teams or both, preferably the consultant, should see parents prior to discharge from hospital. What should be said at this stage will necessarily vary; there will only be so much information parents will be able to take in while in a state of shock. Information will probably need to be repeated, possibly several times, as at such times people often mishear or do not hear all that is said.

As Grace commented, 'More than anything else, I just needed someone to say neither I nor Henry were guilty of our baby's death' [1]. Such a reassurance is a relief and comfort for parents to hear, especially when it comes from a consultant. It is important, however, that parents know they can return to the hospital when they are clear about the kinds of questions they need to ask a doctor. For this reason, it has been found to be beneficial to have an appointment two to three weeks after the loss, as well as the usual six week appointment.

The next crucial time for parents is between two to four months following the loss. Around this time support has often dropped off and many people expect the family to be over their grief. This is a period when community health professionals can be of great support. To have a simple system of phoning or visiting a family may make all the difference to their recovery.

Following discharge from hospital parents should have access to a named person. This may be a nurse on the neonatal unit, a chaplain, social worker or bereavement officer. A well-planned team approach in the hospital caring for families who are bereaved through the death of their baby, should be well supported by a similar team effort in the community, with different professionals being involved as appropriate.

The health professional both in hospital and in the community can help bereaved parents by enabling them to talk freely of their loss and what it means to them. Sometimes a priest or religious adviser knows the family well, and can facilitate a healthy grieving process. If not, it may be the health professional to whom the family turn to provide the kind of support associated with bereavement or other similar trauma.

There can sometimes be quite distressing physical symptoms in acute grief, for instance, tightness in the chest, dry mouth, shortness of breath, and an empty nauseous feeling in the stomach. Occasionally physical symptoms can persist such as headaches and gastrointestinal and sleep disturbances. It is possible these and other severe complaints can be misdiagnosed, especially if a parent is seen by a different doctor some time after the loss of a baby. Those symptoms are then treated, instead of reaching the root cause. This is particularly important to note when it is apparent a person is becoming depressed. Prescribing anti-depressants is not necessarily the wisest course of action, though at times it will be essential. Depression and deep sadness in relation to grief often needs to be experienced in order for the person to reach some sense of resolution. Sometimes the depression will necessitate medication, although often an individual will be much helped by being able to talk to someone about how they feel. This could be a friend, their health visitor, the GP, or a counsellor. Some parents will find it easier to talk with someone they do not know well.

Family and friends may of course be very supportive. Some will know instinctively what to say or do, others will need some guidance. As the SANDS leaflet, 'For Family and Friends' indicates, encouraging people not to avoid the parents, nor to avoid talking of the baby will help. Simply being willing to sit and listen, and not give advice or say thoughtless things like 'At least you have another child' or 'You can have another baby soon' will help considerably. Being prepared to be available for some time after a baby has died, and not expecting parents to 'get over it' in a few weeks will also be a great relief for the couple.

Very often the people who can provide the most appropriate everyday support are those who have experienced a similar loss. Professionals have a responsibility to ensure that parents have access to support organizations, and should encourage or even help with contact as necessary.

For example, SANDS, a national self-help organization, offers assistance to parents by providing a telephone support service and by befriending. Befrienders are people who have lost a baby in the past themselves. Over the years since SANDS began in the early 1970s, many parents have found great support though the national network of groups and individuals. As already mentioned, SANDS also publishes helpful written information for both parents and professionals. Prior to around 20 weeks' gestation (this varies from individual to individual), it may be that the Miscarriage Association information offering possible group or individual support would be more appropriate. Likewise information from Support After Termination for Abnormality (SATFA) should be available to parents following termination.

THE FAMILY

When a baby dies, it is not only the parents who are affected: children, grandparents and other close family and friends are all part of a couple's network. Asking parents about others in the family is part of caring for them and finding out likely levels of support as not everyone is part of a supportive structure. This is as true following a miscarriage, termination for abnormality, stillbirth and neonatal death. Everyone, including family, friends and professionals, will experience some sense of helplessness in the face of the inevitable or actual loss of a child.

The family may look to the professionals for some containment of their seemingly out of control feelings. When at times they fear they are 'going crazy', for staff to be able to reassure parents and others in the family that their feelings are a normal response to loss can be a tremendous relief.

The father

In some instances soon after the delivery it is clear that the baby will not live long. If there has been an emergency Caesarean section the mother may still be recovering from an anaesthetic when the news is broken to the father. He bears the full weight of that news at a time when he and his wife or partner are unable to console one another.

Writing on 'How fathers perceive perinatal death', Judith Page Lieberman and Cynthia B. Hughes say:

> Many of the fathers were caught between their grief and the needs of their wives. One father said: 'It was overwhelming – more than I could handle. So much to do. Enormous responsibility. I had to help my wife with the labour. I had to help find nurses [midwives] to take care of the problems. I had to phone the relatives and tell them ... I was a wreck when she was not looking [8].

It is often left to the father to tell other members of the family what has happened. At a time when everyone is upset, he may be the recipient of much displaced anger when he himself is needing support.

If the baby has to be transferred to another hospital the father may feel torn as to whether to stay with his partner, or go with their child. Whatever he decides, it is most important that as soon as the mother is fit enough, she is transferred to be with her baby, in order that the family can be together.

It may be that the father is the only family member who sees the baby alive if the baby lives a very short time. He is then the one who breaks the news to his partner when she recovers from the anaesthetic.

It is not uncommon for the father himself, family relatives, and even health professionals to expect the father to cope and 'be strong' at such a time. This may be inevitable in the short term, though the potential dangers in this should be kept in mind as the longer-term adjustments occur. Offering follow-up care to both partners can help to redress the balance when inevitably much of the attention has been focused on the mother.

Other children

If there are other children in the family it is important they also are included. One way parents may want to cope with their own grief is to protect their offspring by suppressing facts concerning the pregnancy and delivery, with the consequence that the lost baby becomes a secret in the family. This family taboo can cause immense problems in years to come and can be avoided by encouraging involvement of all concerned, whatever their ages.

Children of different ages perceive death in different ways. They will often accept a simple explanation such as 'The baby died because she did not grow properly'. They can often cope with their parents' sadness better than adults imagine, as long as they are told, and know, that they are loved, and that mummy and daddy will feel less sad as time goes on. Children may also need assurance that the baby's death was not as a result of anything anyone did to the baby, including themselves.

If going to a funeral or visiting a grave can be presented as normal following a death, children will usually take things in their stride. Again, the inclusion and involvement of children will reduce the possibility of the baby's death becoming a taboo.

Sometimes parents experience a confusion of feelings about their other children. They can feel over-protective, supposing something awful will happen to take them away; or they can feel resentful towards the children's demands when all they want to do is give attention to their own feelings about the lost baby.

It is not uncommon for children to develop minor ailments that necessitate extra attention from parents, or even visits to the GP. This is more likely to happen if a child has not been able, or allowed to express his feelings towards the lost sibling. Helping the child to draw, paint, write, talk or play out his feelings may mean that his distress is expressed rather than somatized. The health visitor or GP can be instrumental in facilitating this.

The grandparents

Grandparents have to cope with the loss of their grandchild as well as watch their own child suffer. They often feel helpless, and may be forgotten, with attention focused mainly on the parents, while they can feel isolated and without anyone to talk to themselves. It can be the grandparents who take on the anger for the family, which may result in their directing complaints, verbal and written, at the hospital.

They feel protective of their son or daughter and frustrated with their own helplessness. They may also feel a sense of guilt, wondering if they have passed on 'faulty genes' and that really they are to blame. Grandparents also need time and space to talk about how they feel, their lost hopes and dreams.

There can often be a difficulty with knowing how much a grandparent would like to be involved and how much the parent actually wants them involved. It may be that the health professional, without becoming embroiled in possibly complicated family dynamics, can help facilitate some reconciliation. This may simply be by acknowledging with the family that each person involved will respond differently and have their own ways of coping.

The grandparents may be further helped by having the opportunity to read the leaflet written by other grandparents, produced by SANDS.

THE NEXT PREGNANCY

Thoughts of a next pregnancy will be immediate for some women and abhorrent to others. The father of the baby who has died will probably be ready to try again much sooner than the mother. Clearly it is helpful if a couple can talk about this and understand each other's feelings and concerns.

The question 'When can we have another baby?' often arises while the woman is still in hospital. Bereaved parents can become very confused with the sometimes conflicting advice they receive to this question. They will be most helped by being encouraged to talk together about their feelings concerning another pregnancy, and indeed waiting until they **both** feel ready to try again. Giving information to parents from a medical perspective as well as indicating how other parents have been helped, can save them from rushing too soon into another pregnancy. They can sometimes find they feel ambivalent about beginning again, because they did not have time to say 'goodbye' to the last baby. It will also be helpful to parents to suggest they may not want to be pregnant at exactly the same time of the year as before, as feelings about different babies can become confused, and painful reminders associated with the time of the year may re-emerge.

Each couple is different, and there are no hard and fast rules. Obviously if the mother was ill during the last pregnancy or had a Caesarean section, she should be encouraged to talk to her obstetrician or GP before trying for another baby. Those couples with no other children may feel they want to try again sooner than those who already have a family.

It is not unusual for there to be changes, and sometimes difficulties, in a couple's sexual relationship after the birth of a live healthy baby.

This can become more complex if a baby has died. It is often the woman who particularly feels guilty at resuming a pleasurable activity. Enjoying a sexual relationship and mourning may feel incompatible for either or both partners. Sex can become automatically equated with another pregnancy whether or not contraception is being used. If pregnancy is feared or just not wanted, these feelings can also be transferred to the sexual relationship. The sense of guilt almost inevitably leads to tensions as a couple will feel differently and not necessarily understand the other's viewpoint.

If health professionals, and perhaps particularly a GP, can demonstrate both that they are aware there could be problems, and be prepared to allow the couple to talk, much of the tension can be alleviated. There will be occasions when referral on to another professional would be the most appropriate course to take. This may be to a counsellor, family therapist or possibly a psychosexual counsellor. Even when sexual relations have resumed, there can sometimes be a delay in becoming pregnant. Obviously if this continues, a referral to a fertility clinic may be necessary. However, it may be just as helpful to allow the couple some time, and possibly explore relaxation methods, as conception may be delayed due to tension and anxiety.

When a woman is pregnant again she and her partner are likely to be pleased and worried at the same time. Awareness and acceptance by the health professionals that parents are likely to experience all sorts of fears, some quite irrational, will help the couple through the pregnancy and birth.

Returning to the hospital and unit where a previous baby has died can be distressing. Parents will feel much more reassured if health professionals acknowledge the difficulty and make allowances as necessary. Being told briskly that 'there's nothing wrong this time and of course you don't need another scan' is less helpful than sitting down and spending a few moments explaining how it is that all is well, and why a scan may not be necessary.

The labour may also be a worrying time for parents, especially if it was during the previous labour that things began to go wrong. Midwives and obstetricians will need to be tolerant and understanding if there are more questions and concerns than usual. Even after the safe delivery of a healthy baby it cannot be assumed that parents will be delighted. Feelings can again be complicated. When a couple have lost a baby they can be both happy and sad as memories are re-awakened. Sometimes they feel guilty for growing to love the new baby so much, feeling they are being disloyal to the one that died. Parents will be reassured to know that this is a normal process and that given time each baby will have its own place in the family.

HEALTH PROFESSIONALS

While there is some acknowledgement that parents who lose a baby during a pregnancy or soon afterwards will experience sadness, guilt and anger, there is not necessarily the recognition of the effect on staff caring for women and their partners at such a time. Breaking bad news sensitively one moment, and being present at the birth of a healthy baby the next requires emotional gymnastics from the health professional.

Inevitably professionals can feel distressed when a baby dies. If they are reminded of their own experiences of loss, which may be recent or unresolved, they will probably find it particularly hard to cope. Caring for dying babies and their families is emotionally demanding and if there are other work pressures, health professionals can feel exhausted and unable to be supportive to parents. This can lead to feelings of guilt, which compound an overall sense of having failed because they have also been unable to save the baby.

If both hospital and community personnel can develop a team approach to caring for bereaved parents, the burden will not need to lie on the shoulders of any one individual. With an identified person to co-ordinate care, it does not mean that the individual personally provides all the care needed, simply that it is their responsibility to ensure the family receives both the information and support they require. Health professionals, and perhaps particularly medical personnel, are also expected to provide answers when sometimes there just are none. This can be a heavy burden on doctors as parents look to them for reassurance that 'this won't happen again'. It can be tempting to retreat into lengthy explanations as to statistical evidence, rather than being able to contain the parents' feelings of anger, guilt and helplessness. This can be particularly true of the follow-up appointment. In a busy clinic or surgery it is very difficult to allow the space needed to explore feelings as well as facts. The 6 week postnatal examination should allow time for discussion, both of what has happened including any results available, and also possible future pregnancies.

For health professionals in any setting, what cannot be avoided is that caring for people who are in acute grief often means living with uncomfortable feelings of helplessness within themselves. Bowlby writes 'Loss of a loved person is one of the most intensely painful experiences any human being can suffer, and not only is it painful to experience but it is also painful to witness, if only because we are so impotent to help' [9].

In a recent study [10], it was found that nurses and doctors were unable to stay with bereaved relatives in accident and emergency departments for more than an average of 10–12 and 3 minutes respectively. Discomfort may cause the health professionals to withdraw at a time when they are most needed.

Parkes writes:

Pain is inevitable in such a case and cannot be avoided. It seems from the awareness of both parties that neither can give the other what he wants. The helper cannot bring back the person who's dead, and the bereaved person cannot gratify the helper by seeming helped [11].

If those caring for families who have lost a baby can acknowledge some of their own difficult feelings, it is less likely that parents will feel unheard or misunderstood. Some units in hospitals have found it helpful to have regular meetings for support for staff working in this area. In order to prevent either an individual or a unit becoming sick (diseased), and less efficient, some means of extra care for health professionals should be established.

SUMMARY

In her book *Necessary Losses* Judith Viorst writes:

Loss at an early age can make it harder for us to negotiate future encounters with separation and loss. But even those who are spared major losses in their growing-up years may never really get over the death of a child. Parents living today in this modern industrial world expect their sons and daughters to survive them. The death of a child is perceived as a death out of season, a monstrosity, an outrage against the natural order of things [12].

It has been seen that the death of a baby, both prenatally and in the neonatal period, evokes comparable reactions in parents and requires a concerted and planned team response on the part of the health professionals.

The loss of a baby is not an isolated event, but will have implications not only for the couple's feelings about a future pregnancy, but also for the whole family. An appreciation of this is a crucial element in providing good care both before and after the actual death. Where hospital and community staff are so deeply involved and affected, failure to meet their own need for support will directly affect the quality of care given to grieving parents and their families.

Towards the end of the twentieth century in the affluent countries of the world we remain shocked at the death of a baby. There are times when no amount of technology or expertise can prevent the tragedy. Powerful feelings are evoked in parents, their families and health professionals alike. Finding ways of acknowledging and allowing the confusion of feelings in all those concerned will move us towards a more wholesome and sensitive way of coping with the death of a small baby.

REFERENCES

1. Cox, A.J. (1986) Aunt Grace can't have babies. *Journal of Religion and Health*, 25(1), 73–85.
2. Borg, S. and Lasker, J. (1982) *When Pregnancy Fails: Families Coping with Miscarriage, Stillbirth and Infant Death*. Beacon Press, Boston, Mass.
3. Cummings, David D. (1984) The effects of miscarriage on a man. *First Aid: A Journal of Crisis Intervention*, 1.
4. Grubb-Phillips, C.A. (1988) Intrauterine fetal death: the maternal bereavement experience. *Journal of Perinatal and Neonatal Nursing*, 2(2), 34–44.
5. Moulder, C. (1991) *Miscarriages: Women's Experiences and Needs*. Pandora Press, London.
6. Support after Termination for Abnormality (1990) *A Parents' Handbook*. SATFA, London.
7. Stillbirth and Neonatal Death Society (1991) Guidelines for Professionals. SANDS, London.
8. Page Lieberman, J. and Hughes, C.B. (1990) How fathers perceive perinatal death. *American Journal of Maternal Child Nursing*, 15(5), 320–3.
9. Bowlby, J. (1980) *Attachment and Loss*, Vol. 3. Pelican Books, Harmondsworth, Middx.
10. Wright, A., Cousins, J. and Upward, J. (1988) *Matters of Death and Life: A Study of Bereavement Support in NHS Hospitals in England*. King's Fund, London.
11. Parkes, C.M. (1972) *Bereavement*. Tavistock Publications, London.
12. Viorst, J. (1986) *Necessary Losses*. Simon and Schuster, London.

FURTHER READING

Jolly, June (1987) *Missed Beginnings: Death before Life has been Established*, Austin Cornish Ltd, in association with the Lisa Sainsbury Foundation, London.
Kohner, Nancy and Henley, Alix (1991) *When a Baby Dies: The Experience of Late Miscarriage, Stillbirth and Neonatal Death*, Pandora Press, London.
Panuthos, Claudia and Romeo, Catherine (1984) *Ended Beginnings: Healing Childbearing Losses*, Bergin and Garvey, South Hadley, Mass.
Sarnott Schiff, Harriet (1979) *The Bereaved Parent*, Souvenir Press, London.
Worden, William J. (1987) *Grief Counselling and Grief Therapy*, Tavistock Publications, London.

CHAPTER 13

The death of a twin

Elizabeth Bryan

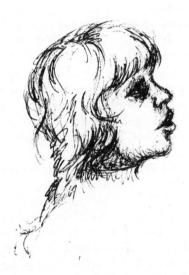

Most of the 16,000 or so twins born in the UK each year will live a full and healthy life but the number who die in their first ten years is inevitably higher than with single children. Many more twins are born prematurely and the risk of a twin dying at or soon after birth is about five times greater than that of a single baby. Moreover the greater the number of babies in a multiple pregnancy, the greater is the risk of miscarriage or very premature birth.

In many ways the death of a baby or child who happens to be a twin is, of course, no different from the death of any other child. But there are some aspects of the bereavement, both for the parents and for the surviving child, which deserve special attention. For example, the feelings of a child who has never previously known life without a partner can be deeply disturbing as can those of parents whose loss is underestimated.

All too often friends and even professional carers may say to a bereaved couple 'How lucky that you still have one lovely baby!' or 'Well, it would have been hard to cope with two!'. No other mother or father would be expected to find comfort from the death of one of their children in the survival of another one. Parents who have lost a twin baby are sometimes even made to feel they have been somehow ungrateful for their surviving child and should be guilty in feeling or showing their grief.

Many people seem to suggest that, because the babies are of the same age one twin should be dispensable or the other at least a sufficient replacement. Yet each baby is, of course, a complete and precious being in itself. It is well known that if a mother becomes pregnant again very soon after she has had a stillborn baby she may emotionally confuse the two babies, the dead one and the new live one. Twinship can provide an extreme example of this confusion when one of the babies dies before birth, or soon after. The mother is then faced with the unenviable psychological task of mourning the death of one baby while she celebrates the life of the healthy survivor. Faced with this impossibly complex combination of emotions, many mothers postpone their mourning. They will then find their grief even harder to cope with when it finally emerges, not least because other people may have forgotten the twin and find it even harder to appreciate their grief.

A mother who is not able to grieve sufficiently for her dead baby while nurturing the live one will often feel guilty about her unfinished business. She wants to grieve but cannot find the emotional space for it. One mother came to see me 15 months after the birth of her twins. They had been born 12 weeks early and the second-born died after only a few hours. The other baby was slightly larger at two and a half pounds and survived. Nevertheless she was very ill for many months and had a haemorrhage into her brain and hydrocephalus which required a series of operations to reduce the pressure.

When the baby finally came home at the age of 5 months, she needed a lot of extra care, including physiotherapy twice a day from her mother. The mother's thoughts had now long been filled with concern about her frail child and she realized she had had no time to think about her other daughter. This understandably worried her. She strongly felt the need at least to say a proper goodbye to her. Arrangements were then made for the surviving twin to be looked after so that the mother could go away peacefully for three days and concentrate on the dead child and mourn for her without interruption. Later the grief of course remained but the mother felt much less frustrated and confused.

The opposite situation sometimes occurs where the mother is unable to tear herself away from the dead baby, and may neglect or even reject the live baby. A mother is more likely to respond like this when people prevent her expressing her grief. Her need to talk about the dead baby may be intense and, if she is not allowed to, she may silently idealize her dead 'angel baby'. This may further alienate her from the survivor especially if he is difficult to nurse. In such situations, not surprisingly, there are sometimes cases of child abuse.

Most people find it very hard to talk about death in general, and the death of a baby in particular. Relatives and friends often go to surprising lengths to avoid mentioning it. With the death of a twin this is especially easy as there is the other baby to talk about. Mothers who have lost a twin at birth have found it is quite possible, beyond the delivery room, for the dead baby never to be mentioned again.

Memories and souvenirs can be carefully preserved and even created and these can be of enormous help to parents later on. If a baby is dying it is imperative that parents spend time with their baby for their own sake, not just the baby's. Too often they are encouraged to give all their attention to the healthy baby. Yet they will have many years in which to give their love to him: they may have only hours or days to care for the ill baby. They may well gain lasting comfort from knowing that they gave all the attention and love they could to this baby in the brief time available to them. Moreover, if the mother really gets to know the dying baby she will find it much easier clearly to distinguish the two babies in her mind later. There is otherwise some danger of her thinking of the surviving baby as 'only half a baby' as one mother put it.

Naming a baby is always important but especially in twins. Not only does it make it easier for the parents to distinguish the babies in their thoughts and when they talk about them but for the survivor, later on, it is obviously much easier if he can refer to his brother or sister easily and naturally by name.

Many parents treasure their photographs of their dead baby. These images provide precious mementoes of both the baby and the twinship. If the photograph is not one that the parents feel comfortable showing to their friends, or when it is not possible or appropriate to photograph the babies together, an artist's sketch of the two together may be made from two separate photographs: the memory of the twinship itself may well be important not only to the parents but, much later on, to the surviving twin.

Even where one or both of the twins have died, most parents want to know if they were identical. There are several good reasons why they should want to know. First, it is natural for any parent to want to learn all they can about their babies. Secondly, and not least, it helps them to imagine their dead child. Thirdly, the survivor may well be highly interested as he grows up. Fourthly, all concerned should know the zygosity if the baby has died from a disorder that might be inherited. Lastly, knowing the zygosity will give a clearer idea as to whether the parents are likely to conceive twins again. (Those with fraternal rather than identical twins have a greatly increased chance.)

It is often not recognized that a mother who has had a multiple pregnancy continues to think of herself as a mother of twins (or more) even where one or more has died. Moreover many mothers who had higher order birth, say triplets, deeply resent the labelling of their surviving children as 'twins'. One mother found herself unable to take her two identical boys out of the house because of the inevitable admiring comments on the 'twins' which just painfully reminded her of the dead triplet. Another mother of quads became quite aggressive towards anyone who referred to her surviving two children as twins. Such responses may sound, or be, excessive but they are very powerful and real. The sudden unexplained death of an infant, otherwise called a 'cot death' or 'crib death', also occurs in twins. Indeed, it used to be thought that twins in general were more vulnerable to it than single infants. Recent studies however show that the increased risk is confined to premature and low birthweight twins. If one twin dies unexpectedly the other one is also at an increased risk of doing so during the next month, and especially during the first few days. For this reason as well as for the reassurance of the parents, most doctors would recommend that the surviving twin be admitted to hospital so that they can be kept under close observation. Very occasionally both babies will die at the same time or within a few days of each other. Presumably the same undiagnosed infection has attacked both babies.

The mother who loses a twin suffers no less than a mother who loses a single baby, but she does have the other baby to occupy her time, not just a huge vacuum. The feeding, bathing and nappy changing must go on: there is still a baby who needs her love and will respond to it. Nevertheless, the presence of the other baby may sometimes increase her pain. A mother may pour all her care and love into her surviving son or daughter while still yearning for the lost baby. One mother described a persistent painful aching in her empty right arm.

Twins are no more prone to die in later childhood than single children but when they do, perhaps from cancer or through a road accident, it can be devastating for the surviving twin. The loss of any sibling can be deeply disturbing for the survivors but the special closeness of relations between twins makes for a very special sense of loss. The surviving twin's behaviour at such a time can disrupt family life. In such cases parents may honestly but deeply disagree about the best ways in which to help their unhappy child. It is critical that such families find support and counselling.

Most mothers have ambivalent feelings towards the surviving child whatever his age. Some overprotect, others reject, some do both by turn – perhaps to conceal the rejection from others and indeed from themselves. The mother may idealize the dead twin and forget that he too could sometimes be untidy, naughty and disobedient. She may also feel that the survivor was somehow responsible for the death. Did he take an unfair share of nourishment before he was born? Had he distracted her at the fatal moment? Had he even caused the accident that killed his twin?

Occasionally, of course, one of these things might be true but, even there, where the fault lay is not the point. With identical twins, especially, the parents may of course be haunted by seeing the dead child in the living one. Sometimes the survivor will look distressingly like his dead brother or even adopt some of his dead brother's mannerisms. One mother dreaded washing her 2-year-old's hair because it was then that she most resembled her sister who had died. These recurring reminders of the lost child have sometimes been so painful that mothers have temporarily rejected survivors and devoted their attention to their other children or to quite other matters.

Most fathers are naturally proud of their twins and the loss of one of them can induce the father to reject the survivor as, without his twin, being somehow incomplete. Some such fathers have insisted on removing all photographs of the twins – a problem that is increased if the twins have never been photographed separately – and become quite unable to relate to the surviving child. This is clearly a deeply serious situation for the whole family as well as for the father himself and professional help should be secured as soon as possible. It may already help if the father realizes that the phenomenon is not uncommon and can be remedied, albeit sometimes slowly.

Many painful reminders of the lost twin and of the twinship are bound to arise. At each stage of life like playgroup or school, the parents will long for the companion who should have been there to share the new trials and adventures. Anniversaries such as birthdays are especially difficult: the joyful celebration of the surviving child may conflict with the sad emotions of the parents. Some parents find comfort in lighting an extra candle for the dead twin and later the surviving child may well wish to join in the ceremony. Other parents may choose to set aside a quiet time on significant anniversaries when they can dwell on the memories of the child who died.

To many bereaved parents the sight of another mother with twins may provoke painful feelings of jealousy of which they may be very ashamed. This is particularly difficult for parents who had established friendships at their local twins club before their loss. A mother can, however, be assured that many mothers there will be longing to help even if they do not know at first how to. They want to be in touch, yet fear that their own good fortune may add to the distress. They will usually be delighted if the bereaved couple show they value their help.

THE SURVIVING TWIN

A surviving twin usually feels the loss of his twin brother or sister far more deeply than that of an ordinary sibling. Strangely enough, this is often the case even when the twins have never known each other – when one twin has died at birth or soon after.

There have been many reliable accounts of a remarkably deep feeling of loss, and incompleteness felt by a surviving twin even in people who did not know they were twins. Some have described how they felt lonely and strangely incomplete throughout their childhood. It is not uncommon for mothers to tell a surviving daughter about her dead twin when she first thinks about having children. Several surviving twins have told me of the inexpressible sense of relief they felt when at last their childhood loneliness was explained.

Even though it may sometimes be painful to do it, I think a child should always be told if he was born a twin. He can then ask questions and express his own feelings. He may at first be angry with his parents or with the hospital doctor who 'allowed' his brother or sister to die. He may be angry towards his twin for deserting him or for distressing the family. He may also feel guilt for having survived somehow at the expense of his twin. However, many twins and triplets are proud of their status and continue to treasure their twin relationship and their interest in twins. One 5-year-old girl whose identical twin sister had been stillborn regularly 'talked' to her sister telling her of the happenings of the day.

Teachers at school or playgroup can help bereaved children express their feelings through drawing or play. The alert teacher may indeed be able to give valuable help to a disturbed child provided of course that he or she has been told of the bereavement.

In later childhood death may be due to accident, chronic illness or a sudden infection and, though no more likely than amongst single children, the impact on the survivor can be devastating. If the one who dies has been the 'leader' of the pair, the 'follower' survivor may feel only 'half a person' and will need somehow to absorb the dead twin's strength to carry on. Some African tribes, like the Yoruba, say the spirit of the dead twin has to be preserved if the survivor is to remain whole. Westerners may regard such beliefs as superstitions yet the symbolism may take on a profound meaning to the survivor.

Many survivors feel guilty for being the one chosen to live. The survivor's guilt, of course, is the greater if he feels directly or even indirectly responsible for his twin's death – perhaps from a prank they were involved in together. The survivor may then need much help in coping with his remorse, however irrational.

Younger children have a particular difficulty in understanding the finality of death and cannot believe their brother or sister will never return. One 3-year-old, whose brother had died in hospital six months earlier, insisted on taking some of his toys to the doctor at Christmastime so that they could be given to his twin. A child cannot be prepared for a sudden death, but if the twin has a long terminal illness it is nearly always helpful if the twin, however young, is involved as much as possible in the final stages of the illness, and at the death itself, as well as in the process of mourning. It is much better that he should cry and see his parents and others crying than bottle it all up. Moreoever the unknown and unseen is more frightening and incomprehensible than reality. For a twin this must be particularly important. There are advantages both to the chronically ill child and to his healthy twin of being together through the final weeks. If the healthy twin is sent away to relatives or friends he will feel lonely and rejected, not only by his parents but also by his twin.

It must also be remembered that children need to say goodbye in their own ways. Some will want to make their own suggestions about the funeral arrangements. They may well wish to choose the toys to go in the coffin or the outfit in which their brother or sister is to be dressed. Agreement to these requests, wherever practicable will be of great comfort to the bereaved child and possibly for many years to come.

While struggling to manage their own grief, many parents will find the sometimes disturbing behaviour of the surviving twin especially distressing. One 2½-year-old suddenly lost his identical twin brother from bacterial meningitis. Having previously enjoyed normal speech development as well as an elaborate 'twin language' he became silent. Six weeks later his mother took him to the mirror to point out some dirty marks on his face. His expression lit up for a few seconds only to turn to anguish as he realized the reflection was his own, not his twin's. He refused to go near a mirror again and became increasingly withdrawn and destructive. Nevertheless, with bereavement counselling for the whole family and patience and understanding from their parents, such children almost always find themselves again and become able to talk normally about their dead twin.

Joan Woodward, a psychotherapist in Birmingham whose own identical twin sister died in early childhood, has carefully studied the profound and unique sense of loss felt by many adult single surviving twins. She interviewed over 200 bereaved twins, amongst whom more than one-third had lost their twin during the first six months of life. In some cases she found that the loss had been experienced equally deeply by those who had never consciously known about their twin as by those who had. Some survivors of newborn twins felt, whether justified or not, that their parents blamed them for the death of their twin. When this occurred the effect on the survivor was often serious.

SUPPORT FROM SELF-HELP GROUPS

As already discussed, most parents who have lost a twin continue to think of themselves as parents of twins and of their single surviving child as a twin even where the co-twin was stillborn. For this reason some of the parents continue to join in the activities of their local twins club. Even those who find the contact with twins and their parents painful will often welcome a chance sometimes to share their feelings with other bereaved parents.

For most parents the greatest source of support is likely to be from other parents who have shared a similar experience. The TAMBA Bereavement Support Group has four sections, one for the loss of one newborn twin, a second for the loss of both including miscarriages, a third for cases of sudden unexpected infant death and a fourth for the loss of an older child. Parents in each of these categories are put in touch with each other individually and through a newsletter. The Multiple Births Foundation also holds bereavement clinics where families can have individual appointments with professionals and also most usefully meet together over an informal lunch.

In 1989 the Multiple Births Foundation established a Lone Twin Network which allows bereaved adult twins to be in touch with each other. Members of the network who lost their twin in infancy or childhood also meet members of the TAMBA Bereavement Support Group so that they can understand better the difficulties that their own parents may have faced. Similarly the bereaved parents benefit from learning of the feelings that their surviving child may have in later life.

FURTHER READING

Bryan, E. (1992) *Twins, Triplets and More*, Penguin, Harmondsworth, chs 11, 12, pp. 87–105.
Woodward, J. (1988) The bereaved twin. *Acta Geneticae Medical et Gemellologial*, **37**, 173–80.

CHAPTER 14

The child with HIV/AIDS

Mark Hayter

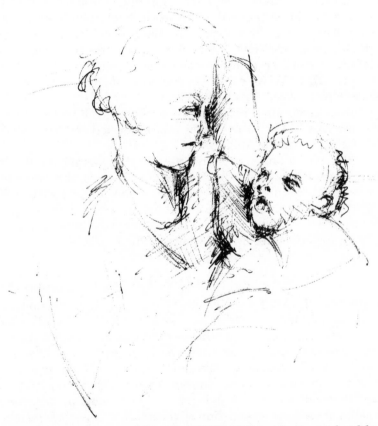

The challenge that world-wide HIV/AIDS presents to health care workers is continually increasing. As the twentieth century draws to a close and the twenty-first begins, we will be presented with a growing number of HIV-infected children and caring for them and their families will require a skilled and sensitive approach. During the early stages of the HIV/AIDS pandemic children represented only a small proportion of those infected with HIV. As more and more women are being infected, and because many of them are of childbearing age, the numbers of infected children will increase.

The cumulative total of women infected with HIV since 1982 in the United Kingdom is 2079. This figure probably underestimates the true figure of sero-prevalance amongst women, however. This is based on an assumption that there are many people infected who have no reason to believe they are and therefore do not have a test [1]. The assumption is made more plausible because there is still a large number of people who present with HIV disease who have not previously been HIV tested.

The cumulative total of AIDS cases in children under 14 years of age in the United Kingdom since 1982 is 86; in addition there have been a further 294 cases of HIV infection in children since 1982 [1].

To realize the impact of HIV infection on children both present and future, however, one has to look at the global perspective. The World Health Organisation (WHO) estimates that, since the beginning of the pandemic, one million children have been infected world wide [2]. By the year 2000, WHO estimates the cumulative total of children infected with HIV will reach 10 million.

To further compound this immense problem, WHO estimates that also by the year 2000 a further 10 million uninfected children will lose one or both parents to AIDS [3].

The HIV/AIDS pandemic is only now entering its second decade, and we must address the range of issues that caring for the family with HIV raises. We cannot wait for medical science to find a cure. Our ability to care is the most important thing we possess in facing the challenge of AIDS. In this chapter I will examine the issues surrounding caring for HIV-infected children and their families.

VECTORS OF TRANSMISSION

Most infants who are infected with HIV acquire the infection from their mothers, often referred to as 'vertical' transmission. The rates of vertical transmission from mother to child vary according to different sources. One of the lowest rates of vertical transmission – 12.9% – was reported by the European Collaborative Study on HIV transmission from mother to child [4]. Other studies report much higher rates than this and there still seems to be a degree of doubt in this area. However, in the area of vertical transmission all the studies agree that the rate of vertical transmission in industrial countries is lower than that of non-industrial countries. (Rates of 13% to 32% in industrialized countries and rates of 25% to 48% in non-industrialized countries) [5]. This variability gives rise to many difficulties for HIV-positive pregnant women who often receive conflicting information about the risk of their child being infected. It would appear that there are many variables that need considering when looking at vertical transmission of HIV.

The health of the mother both before and during pregnancy have been suggested as co-factors for vertical HIV transmission. Prior to the heat treatment of many blood products and the screening of donated blood, some children became infected via this route. While there is still a theoretical risk of HIV transmission from blood transfusion this risk is very small in the United Kingdom.

In many areas of the world however this route still plays a large part in the incidence of HIV infected infants. HIV infection of children as a result of sexual abuse has occurred and obviously adds another dimension to this issue [6]. The risk of breastfeeding by HIV-positive mothers to HIV-negative infants is unclear, although breastfeeding has been implicated as a vector for transmission of HIV, and breastfeeding has been suggested as an important route of transmission [7].

Older children and adolescents face increasing risks of infection as they begin to become sexually active and experiment with drug use.

Routes of HIV infection (infants):
(a) Pre-natally from mother.
(b) Infected blood/blood products.
(c) Breastfeeding.
(d) Sexual abuse.

Routes of HIV infection (older children/adolescents):
(a) Sexual abuse.
(b) Sexual activity.
(c) Drug use.
(d) Blood/blood products.

DIAGNOSIS OF HIV INFECTION IN INFANTS

The diagnosis of HIV infection in infants is fraught with difficulty and uncertainty. In adults the most common way of testing for HIV infection is by performing an HIV antibody test, as the presence of antibody to HIV means infection with the virus has taken place.

Performing an HIV antibody test on a newborn child is of little diagnostic significance, since newborns carry maternal antibodies which will include maternal antibodies to HIV. Since newborn children may carry maternal antibodies for up to 18 months, antibody testing would only be of use after maternal antibodies are lost [4], and an antibody positive test thereafter would indicate active HIV infection.

During this early phase infants who may be infected can be tested to attempt to demonstrate actual viral presence. These tests, however, are more difficult to carry out than antibody testing, more expensive, and some are still in the research phase.

TESTS TO DEMONSTRATE HIV INFECTION

Serological HIV testing in infants

(a) Viral culture.
(b) Complete Western blot.
(c) P24 antigen.
(d) Polymerase chain reaction test (PCR).

Despite the variety of tests available, providing a conclusive result of HIV infection in infants is very often an inexact science. This will mean that a period of maybe 18 months will have to elapse before a reasonable diagnosis can be made, if the child remains clinically well. This period will be one of extreme uncertainty and anxiety for the parent or parents of the child.

Informed parental consent is necessary prior to HIV testing of any sort being carried out on an infant. The lack of certainty about the tests should be fully explained. Testing a child for HIV is an implicit test of the mother's HIV status if the child is positive. Faced with this situation some parents who know that either both of them or the mother is HIV-positive may decide not to have their child tested. This may be done to protect the child from an 'AIDS baby' type stigma. In a well infant this decision should be treated with respect and understanding. Unobtrusive monitoring of the child's clinical condition should be continued. Where the child is clinically ill and HIV disease is suspected the cooperation and consent of the parents to a test should be sought. If the parents still refuse, the paediatrician must decide whether the interests of the child override the wishes of the parents [8].

HIV DISEASE IN CHILDREN

HIV infection is often regarded as a slow infection that causes asymptomatic infection in adults for possibly years without causing illness. This is not the case for many children. Very often in children illness occurs much earlier with HIV infection than in adults. In infants infected from birth 25% develop AIDS within the first year of life, and a further 15% in the second year. For subsequent years the rate of progression to AIDS is around 10% per year [9].

At present the median survival rate for a child with AIDS is three years, although improvements in care and therapy of HIV disease in children will probably be able to increase this in the future. The parents of an HIV-infected child, therefore, may face the physical illness of the child very early after birth. This gives very little time, in many cases, for an HIV diagnosis to be made and for the parents to begin coming to terms with the HIV status of their child. The physiological aspects of HIV disease in children varies quite considerably from that in adults, and is classified in a different manner from adult HIV disease. The Center for Disease Control definitions of HIV and AIDS in children can be seen in Tables 14.1 and 14.2.

Table 14.1 CDC case definition for AIDS in children under 13 years of age

For the limited purposes of epidemiologic surveillance, CDC defines a case of paediatric AIDS as a child under 13 years of age who has had:
1. A reliably diagnosed disease at least moderately indicative of underlying cellular immunodeficiency, *and*
2. No known cause of underlying cellular immunodeficiency or any other reduced resistance reported to be associated with that disease.

The diseases accepted as sufficiently indicative of underlying cellular immunodeficiency are:
candidiasis of the oesophagus, trachea, bronchi or lungs;
cryptococcosis, extrapulmonary;
cryptosporidiosis with diarrhoea persisting for more than 1 month;
cytomegalovirus disease of an organ other than liver, spleen or lymph nodes in a child more than 1month of age;
Herpes simplex virus infection causing a mucocutaneous ulcer that persists longer than 1 month; or bronchitis, pneumonitis or oesophagitis for any duration in a child more than 1 month of age;
lymphoid interstitial pneumonia and/or pulmonary lymphoid hyperplasia (LIP/PLH complex) affecting a child less than 13 years of age;
Mycobacterium avium complex or *M. kansasii* disease, disseminated (at a site other than or in addition to lungs, skin or cervical or hilar lymph nodes);
Pneumocystis carinii pneumonia;
progressive multifocal leucoencephalopathy;
toxoplasmosis of the brain affecting a child more than 1 month of age;
bacterial infections, multiple or recurrent (any combination of at least two within a two-year period), of the following types affecting a child less than 13 years of age:*
    septicaemia, pneumonia, meningitis, bone or joint infection, or abscess of an internal organ or body cavity (excluding otitis media or superficial skin or mucosal abcesses), causes by *Haemophilus, Streptococcus* including *Pneumococcus*), or other pyogenic bacteria;
coccidioidomycosis, disseminated (at a site other than or in addition to lungs, or cervical or hilar lymph nodes);*
HIV encephalopathy;
histoplasmosis, disseminated (at a site other than or in addition to lungs or cervical or hilar lymph nodes);*
isoporiasis with diarrhoea persisting for more than 1 month;*
Kaposi's sarcoma at any age;
lymphoma of the brain (primary) at any age?*
other non-Hodgkin's lymphoma of B cell or unknown immunologic phenotype;*
Specific conditions that must be excluded in a child are:
1. Primary immunodeficiency diseases – severe, combined immuno-deficiency (SCID), DiGeorge syndrome, Wiskott-Aldrich syndrome, ataxia telangiectasia, graft-versus-host disease, neutropenia, neutorphil function abnormality, agammaglobulinaemia, or hypogammaglobulinaemia with raised IgM.
2. Secondary immunodeficiency associated with immunosuppressive therapy, lymphoreticular malignancy or starvation.

*Indicates a diagnosis of AIDS only if there is also laboratory evidence of HIV infection.

Table 14.2 Summary of classification of HIV infection in children less than 13 years of age

Class P-O Indeterminate infection
Class P-1 Asymptomatic infection
Subclass A Normal immune function
Subclass B Abnormal immune function
Subclass C Immune function not tested
Class P-2 Symptomatic infection
Subclass A Nonspecific findings
Subclass B Progressive neurological disease
Subclass C Lymphoid interstitial pneumonitis
Subclass D Secondary infectious diseases
Category D-1 Specified secondary infectious diseases listed in CDC surveillance definition for AIDS
Category D-2 Recurrent serious bacterial infections
Category D-3 Other specified secondary infectious diseases
Subclass E Secondary cancers
Category E-1 Specified secondary cancers listed in CDC surveillance definition for AIDS
Category E-2 Other cancers possibly secondary to HIV infection
Subclass F Other diseases possibly due to HIV infection

The physiological problems that can occur in the HIV-infected child are many and varied, as Table 14.1 shows. Constantly looking for early signs of infection in a child could become obsessive on the part of the parents and it must be stressed that HIV infected children are just as prone to commonplace childhood maladies as uninfected children. Many of the signs of HIV disease are mimicked by these ordinary childhood health problems, such as fever, lymphadenopathy and diarrhoea. The health care worker must be aware that minor symptoms can provoke intense anxiety on the part of the parents and must treat them with care and understanding.

Indication of probable prognosis can be determined from the condition of the child [9]. Signs that often indicate a poor prognosis include:

(a) Early onset of symptoms.
(b) Encephalitis.
(c) Pneumocystis carinii pneumonia.
(d) Anaemia.

Signs that indicate a better prognosis include:

(a) Later onset of symptoms.
(b) AIDS diagnosis over 1 year of age.
(c) Early diagnosis.
(d) Mild symptoms with lymphadenopathy.

AIDS is much more than a disease. Unfortunately, since the onset of the epidemic HIV/AIDS has been surrounded by fear, ignorance, stigma and misinformation. This has led to many people living with HIV or AIDS being confronted, not only with potential or actual ill health, but having to live with widespread prejudice and discrimination. Many of the problems that the parents with an HIV-infected child face are due not to the ill health of the child, but to the way in which HIV infection and AIDS is regarded by society. The health care worker needs to be fully aware of this, and recognize also that some of this prejudice and unfair discrimination occurs within the health care setting as well as without [10]. Usually the parents of an ill child, or a terminally ill child, can expect universal help and compassion. When that child is ill with AIDS, however, in many cases that help and compassion is lacking, and the parents are often seen as being to blame for the child's infection.

AIDS is very often a family unit disease; several of the children and one or both parents may be infected. This adds further dimensions to the difficulties faced by the family and carers, creating a situation that has very few parallels.

ISSUES FOR FAMILIES WITH HIV AND AIDS

Anxiety

For the parent, the realization that the child may be infected with HIV will cause immense anxiety and stress. This may well be, in some cases, compounded by the discovery that they, too, are affected. They may be coming to terms with their own sero-positivity while being uncertain about the status of their child. This leaves parents feeling confused and uncertain.

There are significant gaps in knowledge of childhood HIV, and health care workers may very well be unable to give complete answers to the many questions parents will ask. It is important to be as open and honest as possible, and it is also crucial to understand what real knowledge of HIV infection the parents have. Correcting misconceptions at this stage could prevent more anxiety in the future.

Other emotions

Feelings of guilt, anger and fear are often expressed by parents, and, among other things, can prove to be a significant barrier to communication.

Anger may be directed at each other in terms of 'who infected whom' and possible infidelity in the relationship. Guilt may also be expressed, about having possibly infected the child, and about possible high-risk sexual activity or drug use. These strong emotions in a relationship which has other problems, and is fragile, could lead to the breakdown of that relationship.

The anger may be directed at the health care workers, unit or hospital. In the case of a child with haemophilia who has been infected with contaminated factor VIII this anger could be directed towards the staff who administered it. (Indeed staff may need help to work through their own feelings of guilt about having unknowingly administered HIV to their patients.)

Denial

Parents will sometimes deny the existence of infection in a child. This denial may be their coping mechanism. To push information and results at this stage will often prove counter-productive and serve only to drive a wedge between the health care worker and the family. Being available to discuss issues as they arise, and giving the parents time is paramount in this situation.

Isolation

Strong feelings of isolation may well be experienced by the parents. It is necessary to find out what support family and friends are willing to offer. There is often a strong desire to keep the HIV status of their child a close secret to avoid attracting attention and prejudice. This wish is completely understandable given the way in which society in general views HIV and AIDS. The disclosure of the HIV status of the family could result in a reduction or loss of whatever family support is available.

Confidentiality

The fears expressed by parents about who will be told their child's diagnosis are often well founded. It is important that the health care worker respects this need for confidentiality. The passing on of information concerning the family should at all times be done in consultation and with the permission of the family. All too often breaches of confidentiality have led to horrendous consequences. This can involve verbal and physical aggression towards the family, refusal of services, and social ostracization. However, the wish to keep secret can sometimes hinder care when referrals to agencies are not made because of the fear of breaches of confidentiality [11].

Multiple problems

HIV may be only one additional problem in an already difficult existence. Poverty through unemployment or loss of earnings due to ill health, bad housing, problems because of drug use, difficult relationships and social isolation may compound the problems of ill health. This amount of stress can lead to severe depression which in turn can have a significant impact on the care of the child. It may be appropriate to offer the support of a clinical psychologist. A social worker may be able to help ease financial or housing problems. If drug use is a factor, depression may result in increased or erratic drug use. Liaison with drug agencies would provide additional means of support and help in this case.

Multidisciplinary approach

The diversity of problems that the family can face may mean that many agencies and individuals become involved. There needs to be networking of these various statutory and voluntary organizations, and an agreement made about who should be the key worker for the family. Such a key worker should have a list of people and organizations best placed to help in any given situation.

Infection control issues

Parents, and others, may worry about the risk which the infected child presents. Many of the fears expressed about infection are based on false assumptions. Information about the ways in which HIV can be contracted, and more importantly how HIV *cannot* be contracted, often help to alleviate these fears.

The main focus of care should be to encourage as much normal life as possible for the HIV-infected child, and to avoid his HIV status becoming a barrier.

Basic advice on good hygiene, and how to deal with cuts or grazes can often be provided by the health visitor or the district nurse. It should be stressed to parents that they, and their other children, can cuddle, touch and play with the affected child without any risk of infection.

Many of the 'need to know' arguments put forward by other agencies can be overcome by a policy of universal precautions in areas such as schools, health care, or other communal situations. Treating all people in the same way reduces any infection risk and prevents ostracization of a particular child.

The precautions needed are very simple:

1. The carer should wear gloves when dealing with any active bleeding.
2. Blood-stained disposables should be sent for incineration.
3. Blood stains on clothes or linen should be washed at above 50° centigrade.
4. Blood spills on carpets should be allowed to dry and then cleaned with any commercially available carpet cleaner.
5. Blood spills on other types of flooring or surfaces:
   (a) presept granules; or
   (b) sodium hyperchloride (household bleach) 1 to 10 parts, leave for 20 minutes and wipe with hot soapy water; or
   (c) 70% alcohol leave for 1 hour.

There is no need for the child to use separate toilet facilities unless he has profuse diarrhoea or is bleeding per rectum. In that case he is unlikely to be at school, and in any health care situation it should be possible to provide separate toilet facilities if necessary. At home, the toilet should be cleaned with household bleach after each use, for as long as the bleeding continues.

Children who are infected with HIV or whose status is undetermined will require regular follow-up to assess their condition. Most clinics see children every three to six months, or sometimes more frequently. This provides a point of regular contact with the parents. It is important that the clinic also operates an 'open door' policy, where parents can visit and speak to someone at any time. This is a necessary policy for every service caring for families living with HIV.

Immunization

Immunization has been the subject of intense debate in the past. The Department of Health recommends that all children with HIV can receive inactivated vaccines, such as pertussis and diphtheria, and live vaccines, such as polio, measles, mumps and rubella are recommended for asymptomatic children [12]. The exception to this is the use of BCG vaccination in the United Kingdom, although WHO recommend BCG vaccination should be given to asymptomatic HIV-positive children in areas of high tuberculosis incidence. Tuberculosis is being seen as a second pandemic that is shadowing the spread of HIV.

Health care workers should also be aware of the risk of live polio vaccine to parents who are HIV-positive. Virus from the polio vaccine may persist in the faeces for months. Parents need to ensure that good hygiene and thorough hand washing occurs when changing nappies.

Parents in control

Parents may feel that they are losing control, to a large extent, of their own lives and that of their child. They may see health care workers moving in to take control away from them, and could react against this. It is important, therefore, that key workers with the family establish a relationship of mutual trust. Parents should remain the principal decision-makers, and deliverers of care wherever possible, and must be well supported in doing this.

If parents are ill, every effort should be made to enable them to continue looking after their children as long as possible. Often, help of a practical nature can ease the burden on a parent who may well be extremely lethargic. A multidisciplinary approach, utilizing agencies such as community nursing and social services, will be invaluable. Care should be aimed at keeping the family together.

Ultimately, however, the need for foster care, or more permanent care, of the children may arise. There is a pressing need for local authorities to plan their approach in this problem. They should look at the implications for the fostering and adoption of HIV-infected children [13]. Working with potential foster parents, and covering issues around HIV and AIDS, has been identified as a necessary strategy in reducing problems in placing children [14].

Support groups

While the role of the health care workers in supporting parents is important, the family may gain a lot from meeting others in a similar situation. Support groups can provide invaluable space and opportunity to share thoughts and feelings with others. This is of especial benefit in the field of HIV and AIDS when many people cannot obtain support from other sources. However, support groups do not work for everyone, and while their availability must be made known to parents of an infected child, their attendance is something for them to decide. They should not feel pressured into joining groups on the pretext of following advice.

Talking to the child about HIV and AIDS

Many parents would prefer not to tell their child that he is HIV-positive. However, for most older children, this subject, however difficult, needs to be addressed. The damage caused by a third party relating a child's HIV status to him could be extensive.

What to tell the child is obviously a decision for the parents, but they should be provided with as much advice and support as they need at this time. Information should be given in a way which the child will understand, and it must be remembered that the child's reactions may be very different from those of an adult receiving bad news.

Above all, it is important that the child is not left feeling ashamed or guilty about his condition, or about who he is [15]. A difficult dilemma arises in supporting the child with this information. While stressing that the child is not abnormal, and has nothing to be ashamed of, we are also encouraging the child not to share the information with others. We need to try to explain to him the irrational fears and prejudice which he may meet in others.

NEEDS OF THE INVOLVED HEALTH CARE WORKERS

Training needs

As in any area of health care, there is a need for workers to be well trained. Training should cover areas such as transmission of HIV, infection control, epidemiology and disease processes. There is also a need for those involved to be helped to look at their own attitudes and prejudices, particularly in the areas of sexuality, drug use and life styles. AIDS awareness is very often self-awareness.

Training should be ongoing. In such a fast moving subject regular updates on new information should be available.

The need for support

The rate of staff 'burn out' is very high in the field of caring for people with HIV and AIDS, and therefore any system that can help staff to cope with stress will be of benefit.

Support groups are often regarded as a luxury, or unnecessary. They can, however, be of immense benefit in allowing people a regular opportunity to share with colleagues, and to express their anxieties and problems. As well as regular support, help should be available at any time of particular stress.

Managers need to recognize these benefits and allow time for staff support to take place. Ultimately a better supported team will deliver better patient care.

CONCLUSION

The number of families living with HIV and AIDS will continue to increase. Many of their problems stem not from the infection, or the ill-nesses associated with it, but from the way in which they meet with prejudice and discrimination from society. Hopefully as HIV becomes more widespread it will not carry such a stigma. The advent of AIDS has required us, as health care workers, to examine our attitudes to sex, sexuality, drug use and to different life styles. This may be long overdue.

Being a family unit disease, AIDS has required a multidisciplinary approach and has required many organizations to work closely together. The increasing ability of organizations to do this will result in better care for families living with HIV.

Continuing re-education for all health care workers, and people in allied fields, is essential. This will ensure that standards of care for families living with HIV are maintained and improved. Care for the carers is also an important principle. Giving support to people who are involved in caring for families with HIV will decrease burnout. Staff who feel supported will be more able to work in this stressful area and the standards of care they provide will be better.

Finally, AIDS is a problem for us all. Epidemics flourish in an environment of ignorance and fear. The need for widespread public education and information, and the adoption and continuation of local and national strategies to prevent the spread of HIV, is our only weapon against the epidemic at present, and for the foreseeable future.

REFERENCES

1. Department of Health (1992) Quarterly AIDS statistics. April.
2. World Health Organisation (1992) Press release.
3. International Council of Nurses (1991) Issue, No. 5, July.
4. European Collaborative Study (1991) *Lancet*, **337**, 253–60.
5. Peckham, C. (1992) VIIIth International Conference on AIDS, Amsterdam, The Netherlands, Abstr. poc 4–218.
6. National Institute of Child Health and Human Development (1990) *The New Face of AIDS, a Maternal and Paediatric Epidemic*, US Department of Health and Human Services, Washington, DC.
7. Newell, M.L. (1992) Institute of Child Health, London. Abstract presented at VIIIth International Conference on AIDS, Amsterdam, The Netherlands, Abstr. Thc 1520.
8. Claxton, R. and Harrison, T. (eds) (1991) *Caring for Children with HIV and AIDS*, Edward Arnold, London.
9. Oxtoby, M. (1992) Centre for Disease Control, Paper presented to VIIIth International Conference on AIDS, Amsterdam, The Netherlands.
10. Akinsanya, J. and Rouse, P. (1991) AIDS, who will care? *Nursing Times*, **87**(31).
11. Sherr, L. (1991) *HIV and AIDS in Mother and Babies: a Guide to Counselling*, Blackwell Scientific Publications, Oxford.
12. Mok, J. (1991) The medical management of children with HIV disease, in *Caring for Children with HIV and AIDS* (eds R. Claxton and T. Harrison), Edward Arnold, London.
13. Mok, J. (1987) HIV positive babies. Implications in planning for their future, in *The Implications of AIDS for Children in Care*, British Agencies for Fostering and Adoption, London.
14. Black, A. and Skinner K. (1981) Placement of children at risk of HIV infection, in *The Implications of AIDS for Children in Care*, British Agencies for Fostering and Adoption, London.
15. Kuykendall, J. (1991) Psychological support for families and children affected by HIV, in *Caring for Children with HIV and AIDS* (eds R. Claxton and T. Harrison), Edward Arnold, London.

FURTHER READING

Claxton, R. and Harrison, T. (1991) *Caring for Children with HIV and AIDS*, Edward Arnold, London.
Pratt, R. (1991) *AIDS, A Strategy for Nursing Care*, 3rd edn, Edward Arnold, London.
Sherr, L. (1991) *HIV and AIDS in Mothers and Babies. A Guide to Counselling*, Blackwell Scientific Publication, Oxford.

CHAPTER 15

Sudden death

Celia Hindmarch

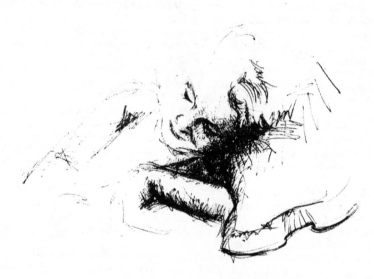

GENERAL CHARACTERISTICS

Any death is a shock to the living. The death of a child from whatever cause is a special outrage. When the death is sudden, there is the added dimension of trauma experienced by the parents, family and carers. Extreme reactions are often frightening, difficult to cope with and leave the carer feeling quite helpless. An understanding of the particular features which characterize sudden death can help to prepare us for the unexpected and to deal with the feelings of helplessness which threaten to prevent our reaching out to those who are suddenly bereaved.

The initial shock, on discovering the death or being told of the death, may be experienced in a variety of ways. Automatic disbelief that such an incomprehensible thing could happen may be so strong as to look like surprising indifference. At the other extreme, the first response may be an alarming outburst of anger or hysteria. Medical assistance may be required for those who react with a physical collapse.

Obviously these various outcomes are relevant to the way in which bad news is communicated. It is not uncommon for parents to be expected to drive to or from hospital when in a state of shock.

Those who are supporting the family after the death need to be aware of the effects of trauma. Trauma literally means the diseased state of the body resulting from a wound or external violence. Indeed, parents whose child has died suddenly will usually experience physical symptoms of their pain, maybe in the heart, or lungs, stomach, head, or in aching limbs. As one mother described it, 'The pain is like major surgery: a large part of me has been cut out. We have to recover gently from it in the same way.' Loss of appetite and sleeplessness may prolong the recovery time. Mentally there is often an extreme sense of disorientation, and fears of insanity are often expressed. The whole system has been violated.

Denial of what has happened is a natural defence against such violation. Disbelief initially helps people to cope, and in the case of sudden death it will take longer for the full impact of the tragedy to sink in. However, if the denial persists for weeks and months, the bereaved person will suffer from extreme anxiety which is likely to perpetuate the psychosomatic symptoms described above, increasing the risk of long-term mental health problems.

Facing reality requires unambiguous explanation and evidence, and ultimately seeing is believing. Only when the facts are faced can the long and gradual adjustment to reality begin and the painful tasks of grieving be tackled. Anger is a natural protest against that reality, and in the case of sudden death it is likely to be extreme and irrational. The need to blame others or oneself may be overwhelming and requires patient understanding. Practical issues such as the autopsy, inquest, criminal and legal proceedings prolong and exacerbate the problem of dealing with these intense feelings of anger, bitterness and guilt.

The apparent randomness of accidental and other sudden deaths adds to the sense of injustice and intensifies the search for meaning. This chance element – 'there but for the grace of God go I' – has special implications. It increases the isolation of the bereaved family and threatens the carers' sense of security. Life can never be completely trusted again.

Accidental death may also involve some element of risk-taking behaviour, either on the part of the child or another person. The carer is again confronted by the fragility of life and may become specially sensitive to the everyday risks which their own children and families face.

Since the death is unexpected, there is no ready network of support, in contrast to most families when a child dies after a long illness. Hospital staff and bereavement support workers will meet the family only at the time of the death or after the death, and have no previous relationship with child or family to draw on. On both sides, therefore, there is a lack of continuity in terms of knowledge and understanding.

Finally, it is important to recognize that unanticipated grief is likely to go on much longer than most people expect and allow for. Coming to terms with a traumatic bereavement will take years rather than months, if at all.

SUDDEN DEATH SITUATIONS

Sudden infant death

Sudden infant death, popularly known as cot death, is the dread of all parents. The death of a healthy baby is so hard to believe that all kinds of myths have arisen which unfairly cast doubt on the care of the baby. This is compounded by the legal requirement of a police interview if the baby has not been seen by a doctor within the previous two days, and sensitive police officers forsake their uniforms and marked cars for this delicate task. There may be discoloration of the baby's face from blood-clotting after the death, resembling bruising, which causes added distress and confusion. In any case the parents are racked by irrational guilt. Did they miss some symptoms? Did they position and cover the baby correctly? Should they have checked the sleeping infant earlier?

In fact, over half of cot death babies have been seen recently by a health professional, since the highest incidence is at 3 months of age when the health visitor is still in regular contact, and the baby may have been taken to the GP with the snuffles or for its first inoculation. Although some babies do have a slight cold beforehand, there are no indicating symptoms and no known cause of sudden infant death. Extensive research has produced many different theories which presently can do no more than point to a coincidence of factors.

The lack of any credible explanation for the death of a healthy baby leaves professionals as well as parents with a heavy sense of responsibility, making it hard to revisit the family and offer support.

Tom was a bonny 9lb baby at birth. At 7 months he developed a chest infection, which the GP treated with antibiotics. A week later, when Tom seemed fully recovered, the family woke one morning to find him still and lifeless in his cot. Tom's distraught parents, Dave and Sue, knew immediately that he was dead. This was confirmed by their GP who was first on the scene. After writing a prescription for Valium, he left with what seemed to the parents like undue haste. They later discovered that he had hurried home to check his 7-month-old baby girl before going to the surgery to look at Tom's notes to see whether he had missed something.

Meanwhile the police had arrived and completed their investigations with sensitivity. Most importantly for Sue, no one tried to take Tom from her arms until she was ready to let him go. After a brief separation, while Sue and Dave followed Tom in the ambulance, though they wish now they had gone with him, they were reunited at the hospital. 'The staff were wonderful,' Sue recalls. 'A nurse brought Tom in to us holding him close, as if he was still alive, treating him with respect. It meant a lot that someone said how beautiful he was, and a couple of the staff sat and cried with us. There was no rush.'

They had to leave him for the post-mortem over the weekend, but were welcomed whenever they returned to hold him again. Tom was home for two days before the funeral, an important time for the parents and for Tom's 6-year-old brother Graeme, who read his book of nursery rhymes to the baby. Dave and Sue thought it best that 3-year-old Michael did not see Tom, but with hindsight now wish they had allowed this, as Michael suffered awful fantasies of what Tom looked like. Fortunately there were photographs to allay his fears.

Sue was left with the overwhelming guilt of knowing that Tom died as she and Dave were sleeping in the same room. 'It took over three years to accept that I couldn't have done anything – and I still find it difficult.'

Road traffic accidents

Road traffic accidents account for the highest incidence of child death. Inexperience as road users makes children and young people specially vulnerable. Twice as many boys as girls are killed on the roads, which presumably reflects a tendency for boys to take more risks and perhaps to be allowed more freedom. Whatever the circumstances, parents are likely to be overwhelmed by feelings of guilt and responsibility, believing that somehow they could have prevented the outcome. The manner of death is brutal and violent. If the child dies as a result of injuries, after hours or days on a life-support machine, the parents are likely to be distanced from their child by all the technology of the intensive care unit. No time for goodbyes, the last words spoken and last actions performed are frozen for all time.

The management of the first hours is important for all concerned. Emergency services personnel, paramedics and hospital casualty staff are trained to deal professionally with this eventuality, but they will be caught up in the trauma and tragedy too. Carers have their own reactions to deal with and need to protect themselves against being overwhelmed in a crisis which calls for professional detachment. Later they will need the support of colleagues and hopefully will receive permission to express their own feelings and reactions.

It is usually the unhappy lot of a police officer to inform parents who were not present at the scene of the accident. Ideally, both parents should be told together and be given the opportunity to go together to the hospital. Too often the mother is 'protected' from an equal share of involvement. Carers should ask themselves: if this was my child, what would I want to do?

Families are plunged headlong into grief. Anger, bitterness and hatred are readily directed towards the driver, the driver of the other vehicle, or the friends who survived. More difficult to express is the anger towards the child who deserted them by being the victim of such needless tragedy. Later, the family will feel further isolated and victimized by a legal system which appears totally inadequate for dealing with their concerns. All too often there is no automatic follow-up from the caring agencies, leaving families to seek their own support.

Other accidental deaths

Deaths from other accidental causes, such as fire, falling, electrocution or drowning, are similarly characterized by a sense of tragedy and parents feeling that they have failed to protect their children from unforeseen dangers. If the physical damage is such that parents are advised not to view the body, they may never come terms with the reality of what has happened, while harbouring nightmarish fantasies. Again, there may be unjustified suspicions of neglect to deal with, and uncertainty about the exact details of what happened. The long wait before the inquest will extend the trauma.

Seventeen-year-old Kevin was a cheerful and popular lad with a sense of fun and adventure. While waiting for the train home one Saturday night, Kevin and his mates explored the goods area of the station and climbed on top of a wagon. Kevin touched the overhead electric wires and was killed outright.

Kevin's mum Betty was called home from her taxi-office job by the news that Kevin had been involved in an accident and found that her husband Kenny had already been taken by the police. She was left in an agony of not knowing what had happened. Her phone enquiries to the local hospitals and police stations all drew a blank. At the railway station Kenny was told, by the British Transport Police, how Kevin had died, and was advised not to see his body. The officer who gave this advice had not seen Kevin himself, but assumed the body to be badly burned. Kenny identified Kevin from his watch and ring.

Back home, Betty's worst fears were confirmed when one of Kevin's friends who had witnessed the accident returned to his home a few doors away. She was angry and distressed to be separated from Kenny at the time they most needed to be together.

On his return, Kenny told Betty what he knew. Two days later their worst fantasies were confirmed by a tabloid newspaper report of the tragedy prefaced by the headline 'Fried Alive . . . '. Before the funeral, the undertaker heard the tentative note in the parents' question: 'Would you advise us to see him?' and suggested they might prefer to remember him as he was when alive. They did not know what they were burying: later, Kenny owned his vision of 'a burnt head of a matchstick'. Betty simply could not believe that Kevin was dead.

Months later the devastating grief which could not be 'realized' began to show in other ways. The two younger girls, aged 8 and 13, presented at casualty with pains and dizzy spells which seemed to have no physical cause, and a consultant referred the family for counselling.

Counselling allowed the family to share their fears and fantasies before addressing their desire to 'know the truth'. First, permission was gained from the coroner's office for the parents to see photographs of Kevin taken immediately after he was killed, photographs that were available to strangers at the inquest but not offered to the parents. To their relief, Kevin was not obviously disfigured but recognizable, and all in one piece. After the relief came the pain and the anger, the need to visit the scene of the accident, write to the papers, and express their feelings to the police and undertaker who had mistakenly tried to protect them.

Three years later Betty was still left with a void: 'If I had seen him, I would have known he was dead, instead of waiting for him to come home, which is what I do.'

Substance misuse

Accidental death by substance misuse carries a special stigma. Experimental use of drugs and other substances is widespread amongst young people, and almost universal where alcohol is concerned. Parents may find it very difficult to come to terms with their child's behaviour, and seek scapegoats to blame. Often the family gets labelled as somehow inadequate.

Suicide

Suicide is perhaps the biggest taboo of all. It is hard to accept that a youngster with all of life's potential before him should choose to end it. What a rejection for the parents who conceived and nurtured that life! Denial is an understandable defence against the burden of guilt and sense of failure which threaten to overwhelm them. Coroners often collude with this and return an open verdict if at all possible in order to spare the family's feelings. In fact the uncertainty which follows an open verdict may hinder the grieving process. As long as the parents can harbour the belief that there may have been a third party, or that an experiment went dreadfully wrong, they will engage all their energies in exploiting every theory which avoids facing reality. In any case the experience of social isolation is likely to be the same, adding a sense of shame to the guilt and responsibility. The stresses on parents and siblings are enormous, and suicidal thoughts of joining the dead youngster are commonly experienced.

During the last three months of his life 20-year-old Simon had lost his job and written off his car. In spite of these setbacks he did not appear to be depressed and his family had no hint beforehand of his suicidal feelings. On a bitterly cold winter's day he waited until his mother took the dogs out for a walk, left a note for his parents, took some rope from the loft and made his way to a park behind a nearby pub. There he hanged himself from a tree in an area where he had played as a young child.

By the time the note was found and the police called, the hanging had been discovered and Simon's body taken to hospital. At first the police said there was still hope of the paramedics reviving him, although they knew he was dead, which later caused much resentment. There was an agonizing two-hour wait before the parents and Simon's two older sisters were allowed to go to the hospital. The police were kind, but when they attempted to talk to Simon's father on his own, Simon's mother felt hurt and demanded not to be left out. The family needed to be together and travelled to the hospital in the same car.

At the hospital the doctor who confirmed the death was cold and detached, and the family wished he had shown some feeling. The nurses were kind and considerate, and the family was given as much time as they wanted with Simon. His older sister was very upset that his feet were not covered by the sheet.

Waiting for the inquest was a dreadful time, even though the suicide note left no doubt of the verdict. The note read: 'Mum and Dad, I did something stupid today, so it is obvious that my brain is not right, or that I am not right. So I have gone to cure it for good. I love you very much, Simon.' Without any other explanation, the perplexed parents were deeply hurt by unfounded stories that Simon had been thrown out of home, that he was on drugs, that he had 'got a girl into trouble'. They felt isolated by the implications that his home and family had been inadequate. The sense of devastation made the family closer and more openly affectionate, which helped Simon's mother through the dark days when she wanted to take all her sleeping pills to be with him. Meeting other mothers with the same experience helped to reduce her feelings of isolation. She is grateful to her GP for his kindness and availability. The fact that his own son had attempted suicide had obviously given him a special understanding of her needs.

Murder

Parents of murder victims are similarly isolated. They are often kept in the dark regarding the progress of criminal investigations, and feel victimized again by a system which gives all the attention to the perpetrator of the crime. They are tormented by private imaginings of their child's final violation and by public ownership of all the details. Anger, bitterness and hatred towards the murderer may be all-consuming and impossible to discharge. For many parents of children who have been murdered, the wounds never heal.

Medical emergency

Some sudden deaths occur in a situation of a medical emergency. The child may have been chronically ill, or facing a routine treatment, when events take an unexpected turn. The death which follows may have to be faced prematurely in the case of terminal illness, or may be the result of a totally unexpected acute condition. Some forms of meningitis, for example, can overwhelm a child within hours, like a supernatural attack from an extraterrestrial force. Family and professionals alike will question the diagnosis, the assessment, the care which the child received and the efforts at resuscitation. The tragedy is that a relatively well child is immediately transformed into an unforeseen life-and-death situation, and the swiftness of fatality renders all the child's carers helpless.

Three-year-old Stacey was admitted to hospital for a routine nose cauterization. Since this was the second such operation, her parents had no anxiety beyond hoping that this one would put an end to the nose bleeds. Dave was working away that day and arranged to phone later to check all was well. Glenda had carried her daughter to theatre and then waited on the ward with Dave's mother. Just half an hour

later they were called to a side room to be told by a doctor that
Stacey had suffered a reaction to the anaesthetic and her heart had
stopped beating – but she had been resuscitated and was in intensive care. Glenda was desperate to be with Stacey but had to
endure an agonizing two-hour wait. She longed for information as
to what was happening but does not remember any explanations
being offered. When she was allowed to see her, Glenda felt
panicked by the machinery and was frightened to touch her at first.
By the time Dave had arrived, a specialist had informed Glenda that
Stacey's heart was enlarged, but Glenda was reassured that Stacey
would be all right.

Within hours, however, Stacey suffered another cardiac arrest
and the emergency team worked desperately to save her. When
all hope had gone, the parents were told that Stacey was dying
and nothing more could be done. The machinery was removed and
Stacey's heart kept beating by hand massage so that Glenda and
Dave could be with her as she died. At first Glenda refused to go
in and remembers thinking, 'If I don't actually see her, it won't be
true'. Dave persuaded her with the words 'Don't let her be on her
own'. They held her until the night sister confirmed 'she's gone
now'. Glenda recalls how she hated her for it, 'I could have done
murder', but knows she needed to hear the words.

The priest who took them home bore the brunt of Dave's anger
at a God who let Stacey die. He is grateful now that the priest
acknowledged his right to be angry and did not reply with platitudes.

The anger and confusion continued after the post-mortem visit
to the consultant failed to make anything clearer to them. How
could an apparently normal child have heart abnormalities which
had gone undetected? They were baffled by the limitations of the
medical profession which could explain the how but not the why.
They obtained their own copy of the post-mortem report from the
coroner and the hospital willingly agreed to their request to see
another consultant to go through Stacey's file with them. They
know now that there are no 'satisfactory' explanations: but it is
vitally important to them that they know anything and everything
that can be known. They are also adamant that they should have
been kept as fully informed as possible, minute by minute and hour
by hour, during Stacey's time in intensive care.

Stacey's unexpected death had a shattering effect on all those
concerned with her care. One of the medical staff involved sought
counselling to come to terms with the irrational but real feelings
of failure and responsibility which resulted from this tragedy.

AT THE TIME OF DEATH

The experience of bereaved families can help to formulate some good
practice guidelines about what to do and say at the time of death.

More importantly, increased awareness can help develop sensitivity, since there is no formula which can be automatically applied to unique human situations. However, it is helpful to bear in mind the general principles to guide us.

The manner of discovering the dead child or the way in which the news of the death is communicated can have a lasting effect and may well determine how parents cope later. The importance of good communication skills and creating the right conditions for breaking bad news is well documented and given proper prominence elsewhere in this book. I would emphasize the need to have the death confirmed by an 'expert'. In the re-telling of their story, parents will often say something like: 'I knew he was dead but I needed the doctor/nurse/ ambulance-driver to say the words before I could believe it was true.'

Following the traumatic **discovery** of the non-breathing child, often witnessed by other children in the family, comes the call to the emergency services. If there is any hope of resuscitation the ambulance personnel and hospital emergency staff will concentrate all their efforts on reviving the child. Later, the parents will need the reassurance that everything humanly possible was done. But parents also need to be involved and informed every step of the way. They have a role to play, however passive. Looking back, it can be crucially important for grieving parents to know that they did the last thing they could possibly do for their child by simply being there. Parents have a right to be there, to travel in the ambulance, to be in the resuscitation room, however distressing or inconvenient, if they wish.

Once this principle is accepted, ways can be found of accommodating difficult situations in order to give parents the opportunity of making these choices. The team can prepare for allowing such options. Someone needs to take responsibility for keeping the parents informed, explaining the conditions and available choices, and if possible staying with them. Some children's hospitals have now adopted the policy of accommodating parents being with their child **at all times**, including resuscitation, if they so wish. This is not easy: it requires a radical rethink of professional attitudes, plus the allocation of a team member to look after the parents. This could be a specially appointed crisis intervention liaison nurse, the chaplain, or someone from a pool of trained volunteers. Other practical issues also need to be addressed. Is there a relatives' room other than the sister's office, and is there space for parents to be with their dead child without compromising the team's readiness for the next crisis? When all hope is gone and the death confirmed, kindly words and gestures from nurses and doctors are valued and long-remembered. Time now for the parents to have unlimited access to their child, to touch and hold for as long as they wish. There will have been no time for considering choices, so in the case of sudden death it is all the more incumbent on carers to inform parents what choices are available to them. Some parents will know exactly what they want, but others will need encouraging reassurance that they **can** hold their child. In such an unreal situation and in a state of shock, parents can be hard put to make decisions, so it is very important to allow time for choices and for reconsideration. A photograph may be declined initially but treasured later. Other family members will want to say their goodbyes, and sometimes parents need reminding of their other children's concerns.

Siblings often later express frustration if they were excluded from the goodbyes. Not all children will want to see their dead brother or sister, or attend the funeral, but I believe that children from a very young age should be given the choice and be trusted to know what they want and what is right for them. It is natural to want to protect children from harsh reality, but their rich imaginations will fantasize what they want to know but are not told, and what they want to see but are denied. The unexpected death of a child is a shattering event for any family, but those families which maximize the involvement of all relevant family members will cope better with each other's grief. Immediate practicalities which have to be faced without any forethought include the registration of the death; the post-mortem; what happens to the child's body between death and funeral; and the funeral itself. One parent may take on the role of the organizer, but if both parents are over-whelmed by shock and extreme emotions then they will need help to think things through. If a doctor has not been in attendance to the child in the previous days before the death, then a coroner's **post-mortem** autopsy is legally required, and this will need to be explained. Some parents want to know what this involves and should be given the permission and opportunity to ask. All parents should be prepared for any differences in the child's appearance after the post-mortem.

Registration has to take place within five days of the death, by the parent(s) or someone who attended the death. This piece of legal red tape is in itself a ritual which further helps to actualize what has happened. Some hospitals may ask for the death to be registered before releasing the body. This is not a legal requirement and should not be allowed to obstruct parents who want to take the body home themselves.

Access is extremely important during the time the child's body is at the hospital. Arrangements need to be in place to accom-modate the family visiting the child for as often and as long as they wish. Again, some parents will need permission and encouragement to exercise their right of access without feeling that they are being a nuisance to the staff.

Taking the body home is an option which should always be offered, as some parents do not know they can ask for this and feel they have lost control of events. In late twentieth-century Britain it may be thought macabre to have the body at home for several days before the funeral, but those families who opt to do so find it helpful and healing. It has been found particularly useful for other children, as they have time and opportunity to get used to the idea of what death means and can reassure themselves that it will not harm them, in spite of the fact that it came so unexpectedly.

Funeral arrangements also serve to help the family face the reality of what has happened. For younger parents this may be their first experience of bereavement and they will need considerable support from family, friends and carers to help them consider options and make their own choices. Induction training should ensure that all hospital care staff know how and where to get the information needed with regard to undertakers, chaplains and ritual requirements of different cultures and faiths.

In the case of accident, suicide and murder, parents are unlikely to witness the death, but are likely to be required to identify the body of their child. Traumatic and brutal as this is, seeing is believing and connects what is told with what is known. Horrific injuries mean that accident and emergency personnel are not only faced with their own reactions but also with the responsibility of deciding whether to protect the parents from the awful and unforgettable reality. This is indeed a heavy responsibility, as families such as Kevin's in the case study above may thus be denied the opportunity to grieve. Taking time to consider and consult with colleagues will give confidence to trusting the parents with sufficient information so that they can take the decision whether to view the body, or how much to view. With sufficient explanation and preparation, most parents will appreciate the opportunity to touch and hold even the smallest part of their child's body. Sensitive use of photographs can also be very helpful.

Sadly, when police and criminal investigations are involved, legal considerations can take precedence over the rights of the parents and needs of the family. Parents are doubly bereaved as the system takes over. Information is at a premium.

In a situation where a parent has been the helpless witness to the child's death, post-traumatic stress disorder may result. Those who have worked with the survivors of tragedies such as Zeebrugge and Hillsborough have found that detailed re-telling of the trauma soon afterwards does help.

AFTER THE DEATH

Six weeks or so after the post-mortem comes the autopsy report. Parents are invited to meet with the relevant consultant to discuss the report and any questions which may arise. In the case of a cot death these questions will often focus on the cause of death and whether the child suffered any pain. There is sometimes a conflict between what the parent understands as the cause of death, for example cot death or sudden infant death syndrome, and what appears on the death certificate from the autopsy report as, for instance, 'acute pneumonia'. This may lead to inflated feelings of guilt: how could anyone fail to recognize pneumonia in a 6-month-old baby? A sensitive social worker or consultant will help the parent bring together understanding of the lay terms and medical terminology. This interpretative exercise begs the question: who is the autopsy report for?

Practically speaking, the tasks of adjustment after a sudden death can be very difficult for all concerned. 'Here today and gone tomorrow' affects the child-minder, playgroup leader, school teacher and playmates, employer and friends as well as family. For parents of older children who have died as a result of an accident it is a source of great comfort to receive messages and visits which affirm the presence and importance of their child's life in the world. Then there is the adjustment to family life: what to do about the suddenly empty cot and pram, the still and silent bedroom, the toys and clothes?

Sudden death intensifies the search for information and meaning to make sense of such a senseless event. Such a search may draw parents towards their religious faith or away from it to a new belief or no belief. Many parents who would not previously have entertained any involvement with spiritualism find themselves visiting a medium in a desperate attempt to make contact with the child they yearn to see and touch again.

For parents whose child has died as a result of an accident, suicide or murder, there is a complex legal system to deal with. So much information is denied to the parents until the inquest that it is common for the parents to maintain some degree of denial before the inquest has taken place. This may take six weeks, six months, or longer. During that waiting time, more attention is likely to have been paid to the 'criminal' or anyone legally implicated with the death than to the dead child's family, which compounds the sense of injustice. Uncertainty about the facts breeds all sorts of fantasies and delays the ability to grieve.

Publicity is an added stress. Parents are often surprised to read reports in the press without warning or permission. The intrusion on private grief can be very upsetting. If the facts are inaccurately reported or sensational language used, there is little chance that the sense of outrage can be redressed. This presents one more hurdle in the painful journey from isolation to facing the world again.

The suddenness of the death makes the task of integrating the past with the present all the harder. The family feels incomplete. If the child was the only one, the parents are left without role and identity. The value of the child's life, however short, needs to be recognized and sustained for the parents and family to live with their loss and face the future. This is where any individual and institution involved with the child's life can help. Parents really appreciate the child's friends calling round and keeping in touch. The school will help the family as well as the child's schoolmates by finding a way of acknowledging the loss. Some schools, in consultation with the family and the pupils, will organize a special ceremony or memorial.

The needs of surviving siblings are notoriously difficult to address. They experience a double loss: the loss of the brother or sister, and the loss of childhood security in the world. They now know that they, too, can die. They may lose, albeit temporarily, the attention of parents devastated by their own grief. Parents are often aware of this but feel powerless to help or even understand what their surviving children are experiencing. Families who cope best seem to be those where the siblings are involved and informed as much as possible, where natural reaction is to protect children from the harsh realities of life and death, and caring professionals can do much to reassure parents about the importance of grieving as a family.

SOURCES OF SUPPORT

In the situation of unexpected death, shocked and disorientated families will rely heavily on the statutory services to guide, advise and support them. Emergency services personnel, hospital accident and emergency staff and social workers are trained and prepared for this eventuality. They know the importance of teamwork and good communication in a high-stress situation. Checklists of procedures with clearly identified roles and responsibilities are helpful to ensure that families are properly informed and involved. This kind of professionalism and preparedness allows for the sensitivity which is also required – the caring word, touch or gesture which is long remembered.

Those with community care roles who are not immediately involved at the time of death may not feel prepared or adequate to deal with the unexpected. The awfulness of the tragedy may be de-skilling and make contact with the bereaved family difficult. Threatened with isolation, the family will appreciate the fact that the GP or health visitor called, that their local minister or social worker visited. Hopefully the extended family, social contacts and friends will provide on-going support for the parents and siblings. However, it is likely that the delayed or complicated grieving which is often a feature of sudden death will demand support over a longer period of time than many friends and relatives can sustain. Contact with other similarly bereaved parents can bring much reassurance, comfort and hope. Self-help support groups like Compassionate Friends and focal points such as the Alder Centre at Liverpool's Alder Hey hospital can provide new networks of support.

For those who feel stuck in their grief, individual counselling or professionally led therapeutic groups may help them to express difficult feelings and re-order shattered lives. For some, telling their story to an empathic but detached outsider brings immediate relief, while others may discover the need to explore issues which take months or years to work through. The availability of suitable professional support is variable and too often depends on the initiative of a particular individual or hospital. There is a case to argue for a co-ordinating role in every health district to act as a reference point for information and support resources in that area.

Whatever the support role, as professional or lay person, the priority is to reach out and make contact with the bereaved family, however inadequate you feel. A mother who lost her baby son in a cot death said years later:

> I shall always be grateful to those who said the right things: I have learnt to forgive those who said the wrong things; I shall never forgive those who said nothing.

CHAPTER 16

Expected death

Lenore Hill

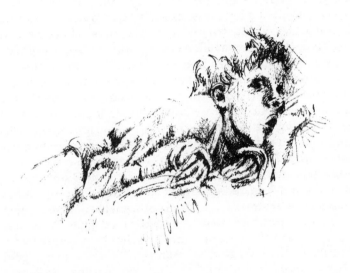

There is a great sense of shock, and many of the emotions of an actual bereavement, for parents who hear that their child has a very serious, life-threatening medical condition. For some there is hope, tied to many potentially difficult decisions about treatment. For others the future holds only a slow deterioration in their child's condition and the inevitability of death. Although each child, each family and each situation is unique, for the vast majority of people faced with this type of diagnosis and prognosis the prospects are devastating. Their child is infinitely precious and they would do anything and pay any price to be able to alter the situation. Their helplessness and inability to alter the course of events is unbearably frustrating.

CHOICES

Some families do have choices about treatment for their child's disease – very often treatments that are distressing and painful and unpleasant.

If surgery is an option it may carry great risks. It may be that initial optimism about treatment slowly gives way to the realization that the disease is not responding to the treatment. New treatments may be offered and more decisions have to be made. One mother said, referring to the therapy her two children were undergoing, 'If they recover completely then one day I may forgive myself for what I have put them through. If they do not, then I never will forgive myself, however long I live.' This clearly illustrates the potential for self-blame, whatever decision parents make. I remember one paediatric surgeon who had infinite patience and great respect for the families he worked with. He always spent a long time explaining in layman's terms, but in considerable detail, illustrating with drawings where necessary, exactly which options were available, surgically, to help the child. He felt that it was very important that all the family were in agreement when a decision about possible surgery was made because of the potential for future guilt and conflict if they were not. Once the family were united in their decision he always made it clear to them that they were accepting the best advice he could offer from his knowledge and experience. His aim was to ensure that any blame attached to the outcome would be directed at him rather than at themselves.

It is important that, whenever possible, the child's own views are taken into account when decisions are taken. If the child is feeling very negative about the treatment, and does not want to cooperate, then the effectiveness of the treatment may well be impaired. I have known situations where once the pressure of compliance has been removed from a child, there has been a change of heart and a willingness to try again. Of course this cannot be guaranteed, and the medical professionals involved will have to be prepared to invest a lot of time and patience in supporting both the child and the parents while decisions are made.30

LITTLE DEATHS

For families who have a child or children with one of the inborn errors of metabolism, or some other progressive disease, there will be no curative treatment to offer. For them there follow many years of 'little deaths'. There is a new twist of the knife with every skill that child loses. Often there is a sudden deterioration causing great alarm, and perhaps the fear that death is now imminent. The child's condition then reaches a plateau at a new, lower level and a new normality settles on the family. They again have to pick up the pieces and learn to care for the child in a different way for the next several months, until the pattern repeats itself.

Most parents during this time are grieving already for the well child they have already lost. Many need someone who is willing to listen to them as they share the past achievements of their 'well child'.

Someone who will look at photographs of school prize day or of the bridesmaid at aunty's wedding. This grieving for their well child is going on alongside the loving, caring and treasuring of the progressively less able sick child, and the dreading of future losses to come.

There are 'little deaths' for parents, too, as they watch the progress of the children of friends and neighbours born around the time of their own child. These children were probably 'competed with' at well baby clinics, and perhaps were at the same playgroups or started school together. Their progress accentuates the regression of their own child who is losing skills as these other children gain new ones. Younger siblings overtake their older brother or sister and may even take on a caring role which would have been more appropriately reversed.

Many parents continue to experience losses after the child has died. They miss the round of applause for their child when he is not there to win a race on sports day. There is the day that would have been his coming of age. Would he have done well in his 'A' levels? This is the year he would have graduated. Would he have had a nice girlfriend by now? He is very missed at his sister's wedding. Would he have married? What of the grandchildren who will never now be born? Of course, these losses after death are the experience of parents however their children have died. They are very hard to share because any concept that most others had of the depth of the loss has long since vanished.

EQUIVOCAL FEELINGS

Perhaps equivocal feelings is too polite an expression for the emotional turmoil which most parents experience over these years. Years of loving, and caring; years of incredible tiredness, joy and sadness, pain and pleasure.

Many parents express positive things about what their child has brought into their lives. A depth of joy and a depth of love they had not known it was possible to experience. A different, and they believe better, set of values for their lives. A depth of friendship and sharing that they do not believe they could have experienced otherwise. The support of other parents and parent support groups; where professional support has been good it is valued as one of the positive experiences. Brothers and sisters may develop a maturity and understanding of the needs of others well beyond their years, and parents are often proud of the supportive and protective attitude of their other children.

Alongside the good, however, is an overwhelming physical and emotional tiredness, perhaps a resentment that the needs of this one child are completely taking over the whole of family life. 'I never expected to be still changing his nappy when he was 14 years old.' 'My house is full of professional people, whose help I need and appreciate, but nonetheless I resent their intrusion on my privacy.' Even to acknowledge for a moment these more negative feelings can bring a great burden of guilt. These huge emotional and physical burdens can put a strain on relationships within the family: between parents who have no resources left for each other, between parents and well children who often feel left out, or pushed out. Sometimes, because their mother is often in hospital with the sick child, the brothers and sisters spend a large part of their childhood with friends, aunts or grandparents. Some children resent the extra responsibilities that they are expected to carry. They may feel embarrassed to have friends in the house in case they do not understand a sibling who may be hyperactive, dribble a lot, have fits or look strange.

FINANCIAL COST

There is a financial burden to add to all the others in caring for a very sick child. Transport to and from hospital, or anywhere else that the child or parents may wish to go, is a complicated and often costly business. Public transport, expensive in itself, may not be suitable for many children. Taxis may be more appropriate for some, but would still be impossible for heavy children with poor mobility or children in electric wheelchairs. Children who may vomit or bleed may not be welcome passengers! A second family car, perhaps especially adapted, is the only answer for many families.

Special equipment needed to care for the child is not always readily available through health service sources. Special wheelchairs and beds, hoists, bath aids, suction machines and nebulizers are just a few of the items of equipment which families may have to pay for or fund-raise for. In order to accommodate all this equipment houses may have to be extended. Grants may be available for some of this work, but parents often have to find at least part of the cost.

Periods of hospitalization cause extra expense: more travelling expenses for family visits, increased telephone bills, extra money spent on food and treats. Appetite may be poor for many of these children, and tempting appetites with sometimes expensive foods is common.

In most families at least one parent has had to sacrifice a career in order to care for the child. The parent remaining in work may have to give up any overtime opportunities in order to be a support in the family. Needing extra time off because of periods of acute ill health or hospitalization of the child can damage career prospects with some employers, and may lead to dismissal in some cases. Sometimes the second parent has to give up work altogether, or work part time, particularly where more than one child in the family is ill. For single parent families these financial difficulties will be greatly aggravated.

Although many parents dismiss these financial burdens as not being their primary problem, they are an added stress to an already stressed family.

THE DYING ADOLESCENT

Many children with progressive or chronic life-threatening illnesses grow to adolescence, intellectually alert and with changing emotional needs but becoming physically more and more dependent.

Adolescence can be a very daunting time for all concerned, without the added complication for the young person of having to face his own imminent mortality. Because these young people become increasingly physically dependent upon the adults around them, there can be a great tendency to continue to treat them as children. This can deny them even the independence of decision-making and the opportunity to explore issues which are important to them. Their lives can become very limited, with few opportunities to mix with their peer group. People are often afraid of a person they perceive to be different, and invitations to join with the activities of friends after school are often not forthcoming for these young people. It is really worth-while trying to influence this, as teenagers will often rally round in a very supportive way if they are given good information and support. This peer group support can add greatly to the quality of life experienced by the affected youngsters: being 'one of the gang', sharing the latest jokes, exploring their own mortality or sexuality and perhaps, for the lucky few, having a girlfriend or boyfriend. Things taken for granted by most adolescents, but especially precious to those in this particular group.

Sadly, this peer group support is denied to many adolescents in this situation, and the gaps left are somewhat inadequately filled by the professional adults with whom they have relationships. Their 'best friends' turn out to be the doctor, the nurse, the physiotherapist or the ambulance driver.

Some parents struggle hard to achieve a degree of independence for their teenage sons and daughters. Others find it hard to 'let go', not quite trusting that anyone else can really care for their child adequately. As with most young people, many find it easier to talk about the big issues facing them with someone other than their parents. This can be very hurtful to some parents, although many recognize it as a normal stage through which they themselves passed. The pain, of course, is that their child is not growing through this stage to independence. The young person is usually also aware of this, and will often be trying to 'protect' the parents from the pain of listening to thoughts of life and death, loss and sexuality. 'Do not tell my Mum what I have said. She would be really upset if she knew' is not an uncommon thing for other adults to hear.

Adolescence is, of course, normally an exciting time full of dreams for the future. A time of great fun and exploration, pushing out the frontiers, and learning to take on new responsibilities and behave in new ways. It can also be a confusing time. Behaviour which was acceptable last year is now challenged as being childish. 'Grown-up' behaviour may be seen as precocious or 'cheeky'. For the adolescent who has a progressive, terminal disorder and for his parents, there are many added difficulties and pitfalls: a sudden rebellion against treatment in a child who has complied, apparently happily, for years, or an aggressive fury about being 'stuck' in a wheelchair; angry tears of frustration about a situation of increasing physical helplessness and a greater awareness of poor prognosis, coupled with a real desire for future goals and achievements which can never be realized.

We have struggled at Martin House with the challenge of how best to support these young people and their families. Dr Michael Shooter, consultant child psychiatrist in Cardiff, shared with us his belief that all adolescents flip backwards and forwards, behaving sometimes as a child, sometimes as an adult. He feels that those of us involved with young people suffering from terminal disorders must seek sensitively to follow their lead. One moment they may want to be held, cuddled and comforted as a young child would, and the next want to be treated with great respect in an adult-to-adult conversation, demanding straight answers to straight questions. They then revert back into needing more cuddles and comfort. This may be confusing to us, but we must allow them this freedom if they are going to feel safe enough to share their pain with us.

RESPECTING PARENTS AS THE PRINCIPAL CARERS

Almost the entire burden of care for these children falls on the parents, or sometimes one parent. To the outsider it may appear that there is a huge system of support available to these families, in the health service, the social services and the education service. Too often the experience of parents is of an insensitive, inflexible system, totally deaf to their appeals for help. They feel that every ounce of help begrudgingly offered has had to be struggled and fought for. Unless it can be privately funded, necessary equipment may take years to arrive, and then be ill-fitting and inadequate. Help with the physical care of the child and extra washing and household chores may be spasmodic or non-existent, and is very variable throughout the country.

It is important that those of us who seek to be alongside families, offering support to them throughout the illness, death and bereavement, listen to what they are asking of us, and do our best to provide the help requested. One father expressed the belief that families are offered 'take it or leave it packages'. He suspected that if these packages were not accepted by parents the professionals went away to consider how to 'educate them' into wanting what was offered. It is not the responsibility of parents to adapt their needs to our convenience. It is our responsibility to do our best to adapt our services to what they are requesting of us.

Parents invariably know their own children very well. If they have established patterns of care then we must do our best to follow their patterns, if we are entrusted with care for even a short time. Changing the timing of drugs, or the method of feeding, can cause great distress to the child and parents, and may mean that control of symptoms is lost.

As the child's condition deteriorates and decisions must be taken about the appropriateness of, for example, antibiotic therapy or tube feeding, parents' wishes must be respected. They may need information in order to make decisions, but they must in the end be the main decision-makers.

PREPARING FOR DEATH

Parents who know that their child is going to die, do have time to plan how they would like things to be. If the child is able, he, also, may want to make preparations for his own death. He may have finishing tasks he wishes to carry out, plans as to who should have the prized computer, or collection of dolls. Some children want to see particular friends or a favourite grandmother. Some want to talk about who will care for their parents, or may want some input into their own funeral.

There are choices that can be made about where the death should take place and these rightly belong only with the family. The child and the parents may have different views on this, and again it is important for us to hear what is said, and to try to be sure that all members of the family hear each other. If everyone knows why different choices are being made, then it is more likely that an agreement can be reached.

An example would be where the child wants to die at home but the parents prefer to be in hospital or a hospice. The reasons for this may well be an anxiety on the part of the parents in facing, alone, an unknown experience. If the community services or the hospice can provide a member of their team to be with them throughout the last few days, this may well influence the parents' thinking.

It is also important to stress that decisions are not irreversible, and may be changed at any stage. As situations alter different choices may be more appropriate. It is also right for everyone to recognize that in the end things may happen so suddenly that there is no time to carry out previous plans, particularly about where a child should die. If death happens away from home parents should always be offered the choice of taking their child home, at least for a short time, before the funeral.

The physical care of the child after death – what he is to wear, the form of funeral service, burial or cremation, can also be planned and parents should be made aware of the choices open to them.

DEATH

Wherever terminal care takes place, the family must remain in control. The child should be surrounded by those who have loved and cared for him throughout his short life. If family pets are wanted, they should be there. Our responsibility is to make sure that symptoms are as well controlled as we can achieve. If parents wish to control the drugs, change the syringe on the syringe driver, give booster doses, then they should be shown how to do this. This is their experience, and they should be given all the privacy and control they wish to have, with sensitive support available immediately they ask for it.

Death, when it comes, is always sudden, and is a shock even when it has been expected for many months or years. Our experience is that most families value easy access to their child's body over the next few days, saying goodbye, and slowly 'letting go'.

THE UNDERVALUING OF LOSS

For parents whose child has been perceived by others to be a problem there is often very little understanding of the devastating pain of having lost the child. The death can actually be seen by others as a positive thing for the family. The problem has gone away; all members of the family can breathe a sigh of relief and normal life can be resumed.

Most parents, in fact, describe loss in these circumstances in the same traumatic physical terms as other bereaved parents. They have been 'ripped open from head to toe', their child has been 'torn from them', they feel opened up and vulnerable with a wound which they feel will never heal. As well as their huge physical sense of loss, no less real than for any other parent, there is the loss of the whole way of life which has evolved around the totally absorbing needs of their child. The attitude of friends and family who demand that the parents 'pull themselves together and get on with life' is reinforced by a state which withdraws all financial assistance at the moment of death.

SUPPORT FOR THE FUTURE

Because parents do not necessarily grieve in the same way as each other, and because each is emotionally drained by their own grief, it is important for them to have someone to whom they can talk outside of the immediate family. Our experience is that this support is usually needed for two to three years after the death. The siblings also need support, and need to have their pain, confusion and anxieties acknowledged. Too often their needs are ignored. Many parent support groups for specific diseases or those attached to specialist units, as well as the Compassionate Friends, can be a great source of comfort and encouragement.

Parents will never forget the child they bore, cared for and now grieve for. Although a new normality will come for the family, the child or children who have died will always be a part of that. One father expressed the belief that an experience in one's life as large as this makes either a better person or a bitter person. It is important that, as the professionals involved with these families, from their first expressed anxieties about their child until their need for bereavement care is passed, we do not give them just reason for bitterness.

FURTHER READING

Alderson, Priscilla (1990) *Choosing for Children*, Oxford University Press, Oxford.

Baum, J.D., Sister Frances Dominica and Woodward, R.N. (eds) (1991) *Listen, My Child Has a Lot of Living to Do*, Oxford University Press, Oxford.

Cooper, Antonya and Harpin, Valerie (eds) (1991) *This Is Our Child*, Oxford University Press, Oxford.

Exley, Helen (ed.) (1981) *What it's Like to be Me*, Exley Publications, 16 Chalk Hill, Watford, Herts.

CHAPTER 17

Dying from genetic disease

Angus Clarke

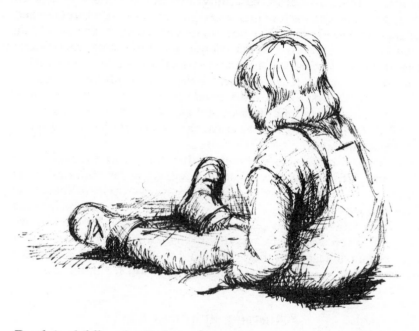

Death in childhood will always bring great sadness, and will always be difficult for families to accept. However, are there special considerations that apply when the death is caused by genetic disease? In this chapter, I give a personal response to this question. This is based upon my experiences, working first in paediatrics and now in medical genetics, and talking with parents about their children with genetic disease.

One important issue concerns the effects of the child's diagnostic label – both the labelling process and the label itself; these may affect the child's identity as a person, with consequences for the quality of the child's life and death. Another issue is the length of time from the presentation or diagnosis of the illness, to the death of the child; this may be many years, during which the life of the family can be dominated by the illness. A third issue is the possible element of rehearsal or repetition in the deaths within a family, when more than one individual has been, or may be, affected by the same disorder.

A fourth issue is that of the feelings of guilt and blame that may arise, either at the personal level within the family, or at the level of 'social responsibility' – based upon notions of (supposed) good citizenship. Such issues of guilt, blame and responsibility are likely to be felt especially powerfully at the time of death of an affected child. Finally, there are practical matters that may arise at the death of children with genetic disorders, that are not so likely to arise when a child dies of a malignancy or from trauma or infection.

There is a great variety of genetic disorders that can cause death in childhood, and it may seem artificial to treat them together as a single entity. In this chapter, however, I concentrate upon the features that genetic diseases have in common, and which distinguish them from non-genetic disorders. I pay less attention to the issues that are common to other causes of death in childhood.

DIAGNOSIS AND IDENTITY

Establishing a diagnosis is of central importance in the life of a child with a possibly lethal genetic disease. This may provide accurate prognostic information, and the family will usually be most concerned to learn all they can about the condition. A knowledge of the diagnosis is also helpful in the medical management of sick children; a firm diagnosis allows appropriate treatment, while avoiding a continued search for underlying causes of the illness. However, the process of diagnostic labelling may arouse strong emotions in the family.

Establishing a diagnosis may bring great relief to the family; they may have known that something was wrong for months or years, but the lack of a diagnosis meant that this was not taken seriously by others. Mothers are told they are over-anxious; failure to take the child to be seen, of course, would later count as evidence of poor mothering: Catch-22 for mothers. A child with Duchenne muscular dystrophy, a sex-linked lethal disorder, whose gait is always thought by his family to have been 'wrong', may not be diagnosed until the age of 4, 5 or even 6 years. To have an explanation for the child's deterioration is of great value to the family in discussions with friends, neighbours, school teachers and social workers. On the other hand, the diagnosis of a lethal genetic disease will always be unwelcome information: it is a high price to pay for the loss of ignorance and uncertainty. This situation will naturally generate strong, but ambivalent, feelings. These feelings will be amplified when more than one child in a sibship is diagnosed as having the same condition. On several occasions, I have made the diagnosis of Duchenne muscular dystrophy in one child in a sibship, and then tested his brother(s) and identified another affected but undiagnosed boy – usually younger, but occasionally older.

One serious problem sometimes associated with diagnostic labelling arises when the child has a genetic condition associated with mental handicap or malformation. A child with Down's syndrome, for example, may then be seen, by those outside the immediate family circle, not so much as first of all a person, who happens to have Down's syndrome, but rather as a case of Down's syndrome who may, subsequently, be acknowledged as a person. A child with leukaemia or meningitis is first of all a child, who happens to have a serious disease. In contrast, the personal identity of a child with mental handicap or a major malformation may be very much wrapped up in, defined by, and indeed limited by, his diagnosis. There are parallels here with the way in which a chauvinist relates to foreigners. All foreigners from one country, or of the same colour, are grouped together and considered as types; sweeping generalizations made about them are thought to constitute a sensible discourse. It is only when the chauvinist meets a range of foreigners from the same country, that the folly of such a narrow view becomes apparent, if the chauvinist's thought processes are not too rigid to permit such an adaptive response to reality.

Of course, the genetic condition itself may limit the individual's abilities and influence his characteristics, but the diagnostic label may add to these biological factors an additional burden of 'disablement'. Labelling is a process intimately related to stigmatization, being most marked for the more 'visible' conditions, and it contributes to the active 'handicapping' of people with disabilities. From this perspective, handicap is something imposed upon people with disabilities by society at large. With diagnoses such as Down's syndrome and spina bifida, it is all too easy for the individual to be regarded as no more than their diagnostic label. In this sense, the individual becomes his label. One child has leukaemia, but, in the brutally honest language of the school yard, another child is a mongol, a cretin or a spastic.

One consequence of the dehumanization of other people, of this treating them as if they were mere objects, can be the expectation of friends and health professionals that the family will not be so very upset at the child's death, because, 'after all, he was only a Mongol'. Naturally, such assumptions may cause tremendous hurt. The value given to the loving of and caring for the child in the past is undermined, and the memory of the child is sullied, by such tacit contempt for those who are excluded from full social acceptance.

INTERVAL FROM DIAGNOSIS TO DEATH

The period of time from establishing a diagnosis to the death of the child may vary enormously. At one extreme, a child with an inborn error of metabolism may appear to be perfectly healthy, and then collapse and die within a few hours. The diagnosis, and even the fact of the disorder being genetic in origin, may not become apparent until long after the child has died. At the other extreme, a child may be diagnosed as having a genetic disorder within a few days of birth, but may not die as a result for many years. For example, a child with Down's syndrome who has an inoperable congenital heart defect may survive for many years; a boy with Duchenne muscular dystrophy may be diagnosed within the first few years of life, but may survive 20 years or more.

It is particularly when the child survives for a number of years beyond the diagnostic labelling process, that the life of the entire family can be moulded around the disease. There are practical reasons for this, and emotional reasons. If the child requires a wheelchair, then many activities will be difficult: holiday travel, shopping, public toilets, going to school etc.; leaving the child alone in the house may be impossible. Similarly, a child who requires feeding by nasogastric tube, or who requires regular chest physiotherapy and is susceptible to infections, will impose considerable restrictions upon the pattern of family life for very practical reasons. However, the fact of the child having a potentially lethal genetic disorder will also frequently produce significant emotional consequences.

Knowing that their child is likely to become progressively more sick and more disabled, parents will often work to ensure that their child has the very best of whatever life is available to him. This may include 'treats' that the family can ill afford, such as foreign travel or computer-operated gadgets, and complementary medicines of uncertain efficacy. This may impose a financial burden on the family, over and above that entailed in the practical coping with the child's condition, and may generate resentment in the healthy brothers and sisters; they may feel that they are neglected and under-appreciated by their parents.

When the child dies, the pattern of family activities will need to be completely re-structured. This can be a major source of stress at what is in any case a very difficult time. The healthy brothers and sisters may feel responsible for the child's death, having perhaps wished for it on a number of occasions. Relief at the death of their brother or sister may then produce strong feelings of guilt. The burden of caring for their child, and their helplessness in the face of the child's suffering, may have resulted in feelings of ambivalence in many parents also, leading on to guilt when their child eventually dies.

The period between diagnosis and death is often much longer in genetic disorders than for other causes of death in childhood. The nearest parallel here would be with death from malignancy, but the hope that the child will be cured is much stronger in the case of many malignancies, whereas the parents of a child with genetic disease often have to live without any such realistic expectation. The child at risk of death from a malignancy is also likely to be evidently unwell, either from the malignancy or from the side-effects of treatment. In contrast, the child destined to die from genetic disease may appear healthy for a number of years, at least on superficial inspection. A child with cystic fibrosis who is currently in a good spell may appear perfectly healthy. A boy in the early stages of Duchenne muscular dystrophy, diagnosed early because of a known family history of the condition, may be developing and progressing at a normal rate. Screening for Duchenne muscular dystrophy amongst newborn male infants may produce similar situations of perfectly 'normal' children being recognized as having a lethal genetic disorder. Again, children diagnosed as having degenerative neurological or metabolic conditions such as Niemann–Pick or Gaucher's disease may, in the early stages, appear too healthy for family members to believe that they have a serious inherited condition.

It is common for families, at least for some members of many families, to seek to deny any serious diagnosis in a child. When the child is said to have a serious, indeed lethal disorder, and yet looks well, this tendency is even stronger. To accept the diagnosis at the emotional level entails the start of the mourning process, and to mourn for a living, healthy-seeming child can be very difficult. In some ways, this resembles the reaction to the diagnosis of mental handicap when parents mourn for their lost perfect child. However, in that situation they will usually have seen evidence of their child's problem. In genetic disease, the factors that have brought the child to medical attention may seem trivial, and quite out of proportion to the seriousness of the diagnosis. It may be only with time, perhaps as the child begins to show the anticipated features of the condition over a period of years, that the family can accept the diagnosis.

In genetic disease, then, the mourning process will very often begin while the child is still alive, and perhaps even fairly healthy. This can affect the family in such a way that every wish of their, still very active, child is regarded as a dying wish that must be honoured. Where the child has only a short time to live, and is ill, then this may be appropriate. However, when the child has many years to live, and is physically and mentally active, this response may be inappropriate. The family may need the opportunity to talk through their feelings in such circumstances. How to balance their desire to love their child, whom they are told is dying, against the need to encourage the proper social and emotional development of that same child, and of any other children in the family. There is also the need to recognize the needs of the parents themselves and the extended family. It may be unhelpful for everyone, including particularly the affected child, to focus so much on the genetic disease that normal life passes the family by for years, and passes the child by for ever. Often, the only way to give the child an experience of normal life, and to allow him to develop emotionally, is for the child not to be favoured but to be treated as normal, to the extent that this is practical. This applies to the time that the child spends in school, as well as at home.

Where the genetic disease causes physical or intellectual problems, for which special educational facilities may be sought, affected children are often grouped together in special schools, or in special classes within ordinary schools. This segregation has advantages and disadvantages, whether or not the cause of the children's segregation is a lethal genetic disease. However, when children who suffer from the same lethal genetic condition are grouped together for education, various emotional consequences can arise. The children's subculture will be aware of their progress towards an early death, even if this is not discussed explicitly with their carers or families. When the child with muscular dystrophy, for example, dies from a chest infection or from cardiomyopathy, then the whole class or even the whole school will be affected. There are parallels here with the experience of cohorts of children undergoing treatment for leukaemia [1]. There are also some parallels with the subculture of the concentration camp inmate, as portrayed in the writings of Primo Levi [2,3].

While an explicit discussion of the issues raised by the death of one of their 'colleagues' may cause the group distress, it may also be a positive experience. It may be emotionally very difficult for the teaching staff to facilitate such discussions, which are then likely to go 'underground'. The difficulty for the staff of coping with these discussions should not be allowed to deny the older children and adolescents the chance to grow emotionally from such openness. It may be helpful for a psychologist or counsellor to spend time with these slowly dying children, either together in a group, or singly, to help them explore and recognize their feelings. To what extent children can be helped by frank discussion with an adult, at an appropriate level of understanding, will be a matter of individual judgement. Such judgement should be as well-informed as possible, and not the expression of unfounded opinions as to what the child or children can or cannot understand [4].

REHEARSAL AND REPETITION

The last paragraphs above raise the topic of this section, the element of rehearsal and repetition that is present when several children are destined to die from the same genetic disorder. The discussion now concentrates upon such deaths within a family, rather than within a school.

Most other causes of death in childhood affect only one child in a family, except road accidents. Deaths from genetic disease are different, in that several children may be affected in the same sibship or extended family. Even where only one child is affected, the fear exists that others might be at risk. Any death will be treated as a possible rehearsal of the future deaths yet to come, and will be compared retrospectively with the previous deaths of affected children in the family.

I have encountered families with two or more children affected by Duchenne muscular dystrophy, by Werdnig–Hoffman disease (infantile spinal muscular atrophy), by lethal inborn errors of metabolism, such as infantile Gaucher's disease, and by a number of other fatal disorders. One lesson I have learned is that every family responds to this theme of rehearsal/repetition in its own, unique fashion.

Some themes, however, can be found in a number of families. Certainly, every difference between the courses of the illness in affected children is likely to be discussed, and, usually, the most favourable interpretation will be put upon the illness of the child who is dying at the present moment. If the illness is more protracted on this occasion, that is a source of relief to the family. John has managed to live a bit longer, and has perhaps gained a bit more and given a bit more than did Jack. On the other hand, if the illness is progressing more rapidly, that is also a cause of relief, because John will not suffer so much as Jack did. If this is the first death in the family, then every detail will be imprinted upon the minds of the parents, and will be used as the basis upon which to anticipate details of future deaths. If a second affected child has already been diagnosed, then there will be a double sadness while the first child dies, as the parents anticipate the death of the second child while experiencing that of the first.

Although the rehearsal/repetition is often thought of as being in the minds of the parents and perhaps of the dying child, it also affects the dying child's brothers and sisters, and the grandparents, aunts and uncles. Where the condition is transmitted as a sex-linked recessive disorder, the sisters and the maternal grandmother and aunts may well be unaffected carriers of the condition. The sisters and aunts of boys dying from Duchenne muscular dystrophy will often be very well aware that they may also have children affected with the same condition in the future.

GUILT

Feelings of guilt and of blame are often aroused in the context of genetic disease. Where one or more children in a family die from such a disorder, these feelings are likely to be especially intense. It is therefore essential for health professionals to avoid making judgements about the wisdom of a family's reproductive decisions in the context of such extreme sensitivity.

Guilt will usually be present in the family as soon as the genetic, inherited nature of the disorder is apparent. Denial may lead the family to look for other possible causes of the child's problem, such as Chernobyl, the mother's diet, local industry etc. Anger may be expressed that the disorder was not detected in the pregnancy, often reflecting the widespread ignorance about the prenatal screening tests applied to so many pregnancies in Britain today. However, guilt is often the most persistent emotional response. Parents feel guilt, particularly the mother if the disorder is sex-linked, or if the child has Down's syndrome, most families assuming falsely that Down's syndrome always 'comes from the woman'. Given that women are still generally expected by their menfolk to take responsibility for reproductive decisions in the family, they may well carry a greater burden of guilt in other situations too, not just in the case of sex-linked disease and Down's syndrome. If the father was reluctant to have the child, or even if he was just neutral, then the mother may well be held 'responsible' for the problem. Even if the language of blame is not employed explicitly, the emotion may well be present. In any case, the mother is likely in practice to have to do most of the coping.

While guilt and blame can be destructive emotions, and can drive a couple apart, there is another possible pattern of adjustment. Some couples respond to the presence of a genetic disorder in their child by coming closer together, and deepening their relationship. Yet other couples battle bravely on, not looking or thinking too far ahead. Perhaps most couples respond in all these ways, positively and negatively. One function of health professionals is to help the family through the bad times. The medical problems may be no worse, but when feelings of guilt and responsibility are weighing heavily, an explicit affirmation of the parents' coping abilities together with an offer of practical assistance may restore or promote the family's ability to cope. The demonstration that the family is not being left to manage on its own, but has the support of at least some social agencies, can be very important.

In addition to the parents, who else feels guilt or blame? The affected individual, if old enough, may be aware of the difficulties that his condition has caused the family. Such issues will often be discussed, along with the question of death, among groups of similarly affected children. Some children can be very angry about their disease, but the response that I have seen most frequently is a straightforward, calm matter-of-fact approach to their lives and to their coming deaths. Of course, this may be because the affected children are sparing my feelings by concealing their own, as so often happens within families too.

There are also the brothers and sisters to be considered. Some may resent the attention heaped upon their unfortunate sibling, and perhaps drift away from their family emotionally; some are wounded because they are not affected too, an example of the 'Survivor Syndrome' – how did I escape, unworthy as I am? Some develop a fierce loyalty towards the affected individual. Some loathe and fear the family disease. Again, many brothers and sisters probably feel a complex mix of these emotions, changing with time.

The grandparents of a child with a lethal genetic disease often suffer feelings of guilt. They may be less busy with the practical coping, and have more opportunity to dwell upon these emotions. I sometimes sense that the older generation feels the guilt more intensely than the parents of the affected children. The grandparents are themselves nearer to death than the parents, and in this way the dying grandchild inappropriately resembles them. Perhaps this leads to strong emotions, especially if the grandparent may have been responsible for transmitting the disorder. In genetic counselling, the collection of blood samples from grandparents can often be helpful in identifying carriers of specific conditions, especially sex-linked disorders.

However, it is often difficult for the parents of an affected child to approach their own parents to ask for this, because of the emotional upset this may trigger in the grandparents. One has to consider the guilt that might be aroused in the grandparents by asking them for a blood sample.

GUILT AND REPRODUCTIVE DECISIONS

How does the question of guilt influence reproductive decisions in families with a child who has a lethal genetic disease? The question of reproductive risk, of how this is understood by at-risk couples, and of how these considerations influence reproductive behaviour, are difficult topics that have not yet received the attention they deserve. There is certainly no simple relationship between the risk, i.e. concerning whether or not to have children, and whether or not to have prenatal diagnostic testing, if it is available, with the option of terminating a fetus likely to be affected by the particular disorder in the family. For the same risk of a child with the same condition, some couples, or women, will take their chance, others will have no pregnancies, and yet others will choose to have prenatal testing, and then to terminate any probably affected pregnancy. Some women will make one decision in one pregnancy, and a different decision in another pregnancy.

It is my impression that the woman generally, but not quite always, makes the decisions concerning prenatal testing. It is clearly right that she should have the last word when the decision affects her body so intimately. These decisions are, inevitably, made on the basis of emotional reaction rather than calm deliberation. A woman at risk of having a child with a sex-linked disorder such as Duchenne muscular dystrophy, may decide that she could not possibly take any appreciable risk of having a son affected in the way her brother had been. She may have spent 10–15 years watching him die, and would feel terrible guilt at bringing another affected boy into the world. On the other hand, she may feel that opting for prenatal testing, and possibly a termination of pregnancy, would be a mark of disrespect to the memory of her dead brother, cheapening their relationship in her heart.

Such tensions cannot be resolved by logical debate, but sensitive exploration of the isues may help the woman or the couple to arrive at their own decision as to what is right for them. It is she/they who will have to live with the outcome of the decision. In such counselling, it is important for professionals to remember the emotional cost of terminating a pregnancy. It is too easy to focus on the sadness there would be if another affected child were born, and to avoid the question of the guilt, lowered self-esteem and social isolation that may follow a termination of pregnancy, even when it is carried out because of a genetic disorder in the fetus.

Particularly if the affected child dies within months of the birth, as often with Werdnig–Hoffman disease, some families express the desire to have another child very soon afterwards. The possible risk that another child might be affected as well, can make the decisions at this time even more difficult.

This discussion has considered the sister of a boy who has died from Duchenne muscular dystrophy, where similar considerations apply to the mother, aunts, nieces and cousins. With autosomal recessive disease, the one in four risk of recurrence in future children is largely restricted to the future brothers and sisters of the affected child, or those already born, so it is only the parents of the dead or dying child who are likely to have to consider the question of prenatal tests in a future pregnancy.

BLAME

Where do we locate the issue of blame in this discussion? We have discussed guilt, which may be regarded as self-blame or internalized blame, but what about blame that is levelled from outside at the family whose child suffers from a serious genetic disease? Surely no one blames the child's parents, do they? Sadly, the answer is that blame is directed at such families, and sometimes by health professionals.

Although the blaming may not relate specifically to the death of the child, it must be discussed because it sets the scene in which first the life and then the death of the child are acted out.

Where prenatal screening tests are available to detect cases of 'fetal abnormality', with the offer of termination for affected pregnancies, some parents may be blamed for having affected children. 'It must be their fault if they have an affected child, because it could have been avoided.' The feeling of possibly being blamed is certainly experienced by many women as a pressure that persuades them to take part in prenatal screening programmes [5]. There is a fear that neighbours, passers-by and even friends and relatives will show little sympathy if a child is born with a 'preventable' genetic disease. Add to this the general lack of confidence that society will help the family to care adequately for a child with mental or physical handicap, and a climate of feeling is created that children with such problems should be hidden away and cared for within the family: 'You chose to have this child, so you look after him.' While such attitudes are not explicitly sanctioned by officialdom, they are present implicitly, within much talk of cutting health care costs through the 'prevention' of genetic and congenital disease [6]. Such attitudes might indeed lead to the 'privatization' of handicap. Children with genetic disease will be regarded as the moral, social and financial responsibility of their parents, especially if the parents 'irresponsibly' opted out of prenatal screening programmes. In a, hopefully remote, nightmare scenario, one could imagine child benefit and tax allowances, maternity leave, even access to health service paediatric facilities, as all being conditional upon adherence to recommended screening programmes for fetal abnormality.

Even in present circumstances, it is not surprising that parents can feel guilt for the birth, for the life and then for the death of their child with a genetic disease. Where a family has already had one affected child, the subsequent birth of a second affected infant can lead to the explicit labelling of the parents as being irresponsible. This may be the view of the wider family and/or the health professionals involved. I have known teenage girls be brought to hospital by their parents for prenatal diagnostic procedures or terminations of pregnancy they did not want, and I have known young couples who have been pressurized by medical staff into having terminations of possibly affected pregnancies on genetic grounds, or sterilization procedures carried out sometimes even on the strength of genetic misinformation. This can result in strong feelings of anger and bitterness towards health professionals, once the woman and her family have the chance to reflect upon what has happened to them. They may have signed a consent form, but they may not have experienced it as giving valid consent.

The doctors who instruct these parents as to what they should do are generally those who refer families for genetic counselling on the understanding that the medical geneticist will reinforce their directives. Those geneticists who do not share this model of what genetic counselling entails, including myself, are doubtless a disappointment to some of our medical colleagues, but fortunately a considerable majority of clinical geneticists in Britain have left such attitudes far behind. As a professional group, we have probably come as far as any in the direction of being client-centred, although there are still some aspects of our services where these issues remain to be clarified [6, 7].

Where prenatal testing is available in pregnancies after the diagnosis of the first affected child in a family, the question of blame arises with even greater force than when it is the first affected child in the family and the only means of 'prevention' would have been prenatal screening for those at population risk of the condition, as opposed to prenatal diagnosis for those pregnancies known to be a greater than population risk. Women who decline the offer of prenatal diagnostic tests can be blamed by doctors, nursing and midwifery staff, their families and by society at large for the subsequent birth of a second affected child. In contrast to this, I believe that the health professionals involved should do all in their power to support such women and their families, and their affected children. To do otherwise is not just ethically unprofessional, but implies that an abstract concept of 'the general good of society' has been elevated in importance over and above our duty to the individual clients and patients whom it is our clear responsibility to serve. This amounts to a eugenicist's agenda, and failure to combat this will add very considerably to the burden of guilt suffered by the families of affected children, as well as to the practical problems that they face.

One further specific matter must be mentioned while we are considering blame for genetic disease: the question of consanguinity. In contrast to much of the rest of mankind, contemporary Western society generally avoids consanguinity, although first-cousin marriages are not prohibited. Because we generally disapprove of the unfamiliar, consanguinity is regarded as a morally dubious practice. The fact that autosomal recessive genetic disorders are encountered more frequently amongst small communities that practise inbreeding has been seized upon by those who wish to discriminate against individuals and groups from different cultures as an 'objective' basis for their prejudice. Such recessive disorders certainly are more frequent amongst some minority ethnic groups in Britain, where they are also more frequent than in the Asian populations from whom the British immigrant groups have been derived. This may be because these communities are smaller, and the degree of consanguinity between potential marriage partners may be greater. It is important to appreciate that marriage, for much of mankind, is a social institution bringing two families into relationships. It is not just a contract between two individuals. Once two families have been brought together in this fashion, it will be natural for there to be a series of marriages between them, and consanguinity may result if this relationship persists over a generation or more. What Western society regards as 'unnatural' is seen by many as the very cement that holds society together. Given the disintegration of so many marriages and families in Britain today, one may wonder what are the grounds for favouring the 'Western' understanding of kinship and marriage.

PRACTICAL ASPECTS OF DEATH FROM GENETIC DISEASE IN CHILDHOOD

There are three practical aspects of death from genetic disease in childhood that I will mention here. First, there may well be a request that medical samples be taken from the child just before or soon after he dies, or that a post-mortem examination be performed. The reasons for such requests may vary. There may be uncertainty as to the precise diagnosis of the child, which warrants clarification. The storing of samples of DNA or of fibroblasts grown in culture from the child's skin may enable prenatal testing of a future pregnancy to be offered, or may permit the genetic basis of the condition in this child to be elucidated in the future. Samples from the child may be able to contribute to research into the condition in question. The condition may be uncommon, so that the doctors involved wish to learn as much as possible about how each child with the condition is affected. These are all thoroughly respectable and laudable purposes that would seem to justify a post-mortem examination or the collection of samples. However, it is the right of any family to refuse permission for such investigations on their child.

Unless there are strong cultural prejudices against such requests, I would generally try to persuade the family to grant permission for such tests to be performed. Although distressing at the time, the thought that even some very small benefit has come from the death of their child may be of some comfort in the future. Furthermore, accurate genetic counselling, and subsequent prenatal diagnosis, depends largely upon the establishment of a full and correct diagnosis. Future members of the family may wish that every effort has been made to refine the diagnosis as much as possible.

Another issue that will often be raised by the death of a child from a genetic disorder is what to say to other members of the family? This question does not arise just at the time of death, but death can bring the matter to attention again. If there is a significant risk of someone else in the family having a child affected with the same condition, then one has to decide what to say to other family members. An attempt to conceal a genetic disease from relatives is unlikely to succeed indefinitely, and may cause great anger and bitterness when it is discovered, particularly if another member of the family has had an affected child in the meantime.

Finally, there is the question of how the family members may reconstruct their social lives once the affected child has died. If there has been a lot of contact with a disease support group for parents and families, then the death of the child may leave a hole that is difficult to fill. As long as the group is supportive, it may be best to continue attending meetings as previously, and only to discontinue this very gradually, as other activities come to claim the time instead. A final coming-to-terms with the death of a child from genetic disease may entail a continued commitment to such a family support group, or it may entail leaving the group. These decisions will be different for everyone. What is important, is for each individual to recognize their own needs, and not to act as they are expected to by others.

REFERENCES

1. Bluebond-Langner, M. (1978) *The Private Worlds of Dying Children*, Princeton University Press, Princeton.
2. Levi, P. (1979) *If This is a Man*, Penguin Books, Harmondsworth.
3. Levi, P. (1979) *The Truce*, Penguin Books, Harmondsworth.
4. Anthony, S. (1971) *The Discovery of Death in Childhood and After*, Allen Lane, London (and Penguin Education, 1973).
5. Lippman, A. (1991) Prenatal genetic testing and screening: constructing needs and reinforcing inequities. *American Journal of Law and Medicine*, **17**, 15–50.
6. Clarke, A. (1990) Genetics, ethics and audit. *Lancet*, **334**, 1145–7.
7. Clarke, A. (1991) Is non-directive genetic counselling possible? *Lancet*, **338**, 998–1001.

FURTHER READING

Boston, S. (1981) *Will My Son: The Life and Death of a Mongol Child*, Pluto Press, London.
Oliver, M. (1990) *The Politics of Disablement*, Macmillan Education, London.

Resources available

This list is not exhaustive. There are many local support agencies available for families.

If you are looking for help in an area not mentioned in this list, please contact either ACT or Contact A Family as they both hold comprehensive information and will be very helpful. For local information on services for children with cancer, contact either Malcolm Sargent Cancer Fund for Children or the nearest paediatric oncology department.

ACT
    Association for Children with Terminal or Life Threatening Conditions and their Families
65 St Michael's Hill
Bristol BS2 8DZ
0272 215411

Exists to provide a national resource for parents and professionals caring for children with terminal and life-threatening conditions. It aims to inform families of available services, both in the statutory and voluntary sectors, through its national database. It supports those planning and providing children's hospices and related services, and organizes national conferences to provide a forum for education and debate.

AIDS
    Positively Women
5 Sebastian Street
London EC1V 0HE
071 490 5515

Provides emotional support to HIV-positive women, including mothers.

Positive Options (Barnardos)
354 Goswell Road
London EC1V 7LQ
071 278 5039

Provides information, advice and support for parents
who are HIV-positive and who need help in making
plans for the future care of their children. The
scheme is confidential and independent.

Terence Higgins Trust
52–54 Grays Inn Road
London WC1X 8JU
071 831 0330

Counselling service in London, information service
nationally. (National helpline 071 242 1010.)

Barnardos   Tanners Lane
Barkingside
Ilford
Essex IG6 1QG
081 550 8822

Barnardos are involved in support for children with
life-threatening disorders in some regional centres.
Contact Information Officer at the above address for
information about any local resources.

Benefits   There are a range of DSS benefits which may be
available for the child or family. Contact local social
security office for advice.

Bereavement   *Compassionate Friends*
53 North Street
Bristol BS3 1EN
0272 539639

National organization offering support to parents
and siblings of children who have died.

Cruse
Cruse House
126 Sheen Road
Richmond
Surrey TN9 1UR
081 940 4818

Offers bereavement care to any bereaved person.
Those wishing to speak directly to a counsellor
should ring 081 332 7227.

Foundation for Study of Infant Death
35 Belgrave Square
London SW1X 8QB
071 235 0965

Information centre for parents and professionals.
Personal support for bereaved families.

Miscarriage Association
c/o Clayton Hospital
Northgate
Wakefield
W. Yorkshire WF1 3JS
0924 200799 (most weekday mornings)

SAFTA
Support After Termination for Abnormality
29–30 Soho Square
London W1V 6JB
071 439 6124
071 287 3753

SANDS
Stillbirth and Neonatal Death Society
28 Portland Place
London W1N 4DE
071 436 5881

Blisslink　　17–21 Emerald Street
London WC1N 3QL
071 831 93993/8996

For parents whose babies are in intensive care units.
Bereaved parents are referred to SANDS.

Cancer　　There are many statutory and voluntary agencies
offering emotional, physical and financial help to
families with a child suffering from cancer. Malcolm

Sargent Cancer Fund for Children or the paediatric oncology unit treating the child will have details of what is available locally.

Malcolm Sargent Cancer Fund For Children
14 Abingdon Road
London W8 6AF
071 937 4548

Counselling, emotional and practical support and information on other local resources, are available to children with cancer (up to age 21) and their families, at all stages of their disease, through Malcolm Sargent Social Workers who are attached to the main children's cancer treatment centres throughout the British Isles.

In some centres there are also Malcolm Sargent Play Therapists and, in Scotland, a Malcolm Sargent Occupational Therapist and a Malcolm Sargent Nurse. The Malcolm Sargent Fund also gives direct financial grants to families, and provides all-year full-board holiday centres at no cost to the child and one carer, and low cost to the rest of the family. Grants and holidays are usually arranged through the Malcolm Sargent Social Worker or other hospital social worker.

Contact a Family

16 Strutton Ground
London SW1P 2HP
071 222 2695

Offers information, advice and support to families or professionals who are caring for a child with any type of disability or special need.

Cystic fibrosis

Cystic Fibrosis Research Trust
Alexandra House
5 Blyth Road
Bromley
Kent BR1 3RS
081 464 7211

Offers support and advice to families throughout the UK. Over 30 local groups. Holiday caravans at nominal charge. Books and booklets available on all aspects of cystic fibrosis (catalogue on request).

Heart care   *Children's Heart Support Federation*
                          17 Cote Lane
                          Mossley
                          Lancs OL15 9DF
                          0457 833585

                          Central contact point for all heart care groups in
                          various parts of the UK. Through the office contact
                          with other parents and support to individual
                          groups.

                          Heart to Heart/Lung Transplant
                          62 Hillmorton Road
                          Rugby
                          Warwickshire CV22 5AF
                          0788 548961

                          Supports families whose children are awaiting or
                          have received heart or heart/lung transplants. Also
                          offers bereavement support for families whose child
                          has died before or after transplantation.

Hospices for   Type of service offered is outlined in Chapter
children   11.

                          Acorns
                          103 Oak Tree Lane
                          Selly Oak
                          Birmingham B29 6HZ
                          021 414 1741

                          Children's Hospice for the Eastern Region
                          Milton
                          Cambridge
                          CB4 4AB
                          0223 860306

                          Francis House
                          390 Parrswood Road
                          Didsbury
                          Manchester M20 09A
                          061 434 4118

Helen House
37 Leopold Street
Oxford OX4 1QT
0865 728251

Martin House
Grove Road
Clifford
Wetherby
W. Yorkshire LS23 6TX
0937 845045

Kidney disease   *British Kidney Patient Association*
Bordon
Hants GU35 9JZ
0420 472021

Offers information and support for families, including some financial support. Offers some holiday provision for children or families.

Liver disease   *Children's Liver Disease Foundation*
138 Digbeth
Birmingham
B5 6DR
021 643 7282

Offers information and support to families whose children suffer from liver disease.

Metabolic
disorders   *MPS Society*
Society for Mucopolysaccharide Disease
7 Chessfield Park
Little Chalfont
Buckinghamshire HP6 6RW
0494 762789

Offers information, support and practical help for families caring for a child with a mucopolysaccharide disorder.

R.T.M.D.C.
The Research Trust for Metabolic Disease in
Children
Golden Gates Lodge
Weston Road
Crewe
Cheshire CW1 1XN
0270 250221

Offers information and support (sometimes
including financial support) for families caring
for children suffering from a metabolic disorder.

Neuromuscular *Jennifer Trust for Spinal Muscular Atrophy*
degenerative 11 Ash Tree Close
disorders Wellesbourne
Warwick CV35 9SA
0789 842377

Emotional and practical support for families whose
children suffer from any of the spinal muscular
atrophies.

Muscular Dystrophy Group of Great Britain & Northern
Ireland
7–11 Prescott Place
London SW4 6BS
071 720 8055

Offers information, emotional, practical and financial help for families. Family care officers based at
Regional centres also offer support to families
whose children suffer from spinal muscular
atrophy.

REACT *Research, Education and Aid for Children with Terminal*
Disease
73 Whitehall Park Road
London W4 3NB
081 995 8188

Assists children with life-threatening disease and
their families when faced with unexpected financial needs. REACT attempts to respond immediately
to applications from parents (through their doctor

or other professional workers). As resources become available REACT will increasingly fund research into the treatment of these children, and the problems faced by their carers.

Twins

Multiple Births Foundation
Queen Charlotte's and Chelsea Hospital
Goldhawk Road
London W6 0XG
081 4666 ext. 5201

Professional support of families with twins and higher multiple births.

TAMBA
Twins and Multiple Births Association
PO Box 30
Little Sutton
South Wirral
L66 1TH
051 348 0020

A national support organization for families, with twins or other multiple births. (Also offers bereavement support and leaflets.)

Index

Page numbers in **bold** refer to the list of support services and addresses. Under the heading 'Archie', subheadings are listed in chronological rather than alphabetical sequence.

5
ω